THE APPLE CIDER VINEGAR
WEIGHT LOSS REVOLUTION

THE APPLE CIDER VINEGAR WEIGHT LOSS REVOLUTION

Transform Your Body and Lose Weight with the ACV Diet

by Jago Holmes, CPT

Copyright © 2023 New Image Fitness Ltd

All rights reserved.

No part of this publication may be reproduced, stored in a retrieval system, or in any form or by any means, without the prior permission in writing of the publisher.

Disclaimer Notice:

To the fullest extent permitted by law, New Image Fitness Limited is providing this written material, its subsidiary elements and its contents on an 'as is' basis and makes no (and expressly disclaims all) representations or warranties of any kind with respect to this written material or its contents including, without limitation, advice and recommendations, warranties or merchantability and fitness for a particular purpose. The information is given for entertainment purposes only.

In addition, New Image Fitness Limited does not represent or warrant that the information accessible via this written material is accurate, complete or current. To the fullest extent permitted by law, New Image Fitness Limited or any of its affiliates, partners, directors, employees or other representatives will not be liable for damages arising out of, or in connection, with the use of this written material.

This is a comprehensive limitation of liability that applies to all damages of any kind, including (without limitation) compensatory, direct, indirect or consequential damages, loss of data, income or profit, loss of or damage to property and claims of third parties.

Interior pages design: Lazar Kackarovski

Printed by CreateSpace, an Amazon.com Company
Available from Amazon.com, CreateSpace.com, and other retail outlets

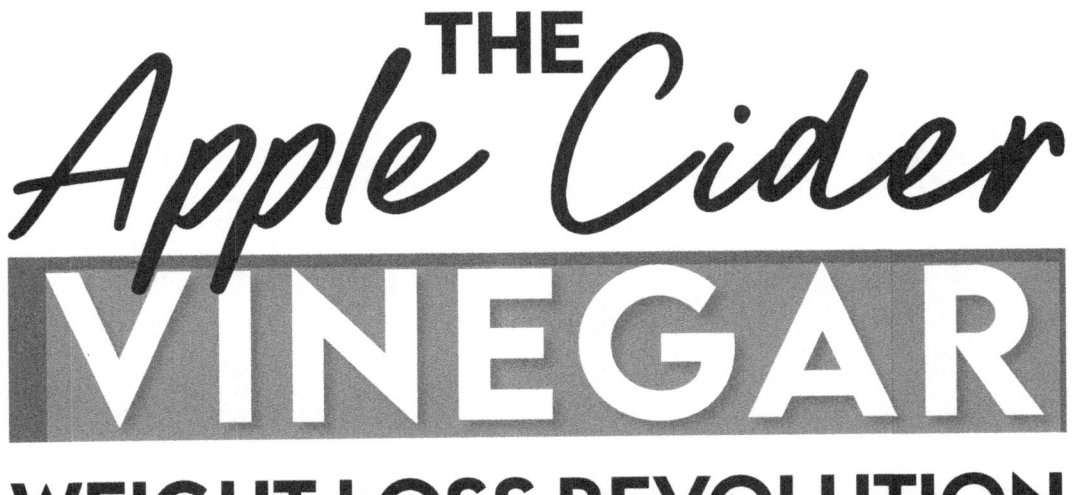

THE Apple Cider VINEGAR WEIGHT LOSS REVOLUTION

TRANSFORM YOUR BODY AND LOSE WEIGHT WITH THE ACV DIET

JAGO HOLMES

TABLE OF CONTENTS

INTRODUCTION 9

WHAT IS APPLE CIDER VINEGAR? 11
Whole Apple Cider Vinegar Recipe 16

The Many Health Benefits of Apple Cider Vinegar 19

Health Problems and Apple Cider Vinegar 23

Common Day to Day Ailments That ACV Can Help 25

How to Choose Apple Cider Vinegar 27

APPLE CIDER VINEGAR FOR WEIGHT LOSS 29

ACV Weight Loss Method 1 34

ACV Weight Loss Method 2 35

ACV Weight Loss Method 3 39

Vegetarian Sample Diet Plan 41

Pescatarian Sample ACV Diet Plan 42

Omnivore Diet ACV Sample Plan 43

10 Golden Rules of Weight Loss 47

Measuring Weight Loss 49

Apple Cider Vinegar Supplements 51

What About Exercise? 53
Basic Walking Plan 63

Walking and Weight Loss – the Facts 65

Using Apple Cider Vinegar in Your Beauty Regime 71

Using Apple Cider Vinegar in the Home 73

APPLE CIDER VINEGAR RECIPES — 76

BREAKFASTS — 77

Sunny Day Smoothie	77
Apple Cider Vinegar Smoothie	78
Apple Cider Vinegar Pancakes	78
Overnight Oats	79
Fruit Salad With Yogurt	80
Crunchy Nut Granola	81
Spinach And Mushroom Frittata	82
Cranberry Zest	83
Healthy Baked Beans With Poached Eggs	84
Ginger Kick Green Smoothie	84

LUNCHES — 85

Indonesian Salad	85
Chicken Stir Fry	86
New Potato Salad	87
Chicken And Bacon Salad	87
Apple Cider Vinegar-Marinated Pork Chops	88
Apple And Butternut Squash Soup	89
Grilled Vegetable Salad	90
Spanish Prawns And Mixed Leaf Salad	91
Tomato, Rocket, And Sugar Snap Pea Salad	92
French Onion Soup	92

DINNERS — 93

Seared Steak With Mushrooms	93
Vegan Burritos	94
Beef Stir Fry	95
Prawn Curry	96
Quick Thai Fishcakes	97
Chicken Strips With Satay Sauce	98
Steamed Salmon With Vegetables And Herbs	98
Bean Goulash	99
Halibut Stew With Cannellini Beans	100
Mediterranean Burger	101

HEALTHY SNACKS — 102

Home Made Hummus	102
Mexican Guacamole	103
Homemade Slaw	104
Onion And Tomato Salsa	104
Spiced Whole-Grain Banana Bread	105
Baked Spiced Pears	106
Low-Fat Apple Cider Vinegar Sorbet	107
Low-Fat Apple Cider Vinegar Cake	107
Apple Cider Vinegar Chocolate Cake	108
Apple Crumble	109
Basic Apple Cider Vinaigrette	110
Honey Mustard Dressing	110

Italian Herb Dressing	111
Rice And Bean Sprout Salad	112
Tomato, Cucumber And Mint Salad With Yogurt Dressing	112
Crab And Papaya Salad	113
Warm Lentil Salad With Parma Ham, Chicken And Rocket	114
Bean, Potato And Tuna Salad	115
Mint Sauce	116
Apple Cider Vinegar Drinks	117

Apple Cider Vinegar Frequently Asked Questions — 119

Book Summary	**123**
About The Author	**124**
Other Books That Might Be of Interest to You	**126**
Useful Forms, Planners and Logs	**127**
Aims and Objectives	127
Weekly Measurements	**129**
How to Use This Form	129
Your Workout Log	130
Activity Planner	132

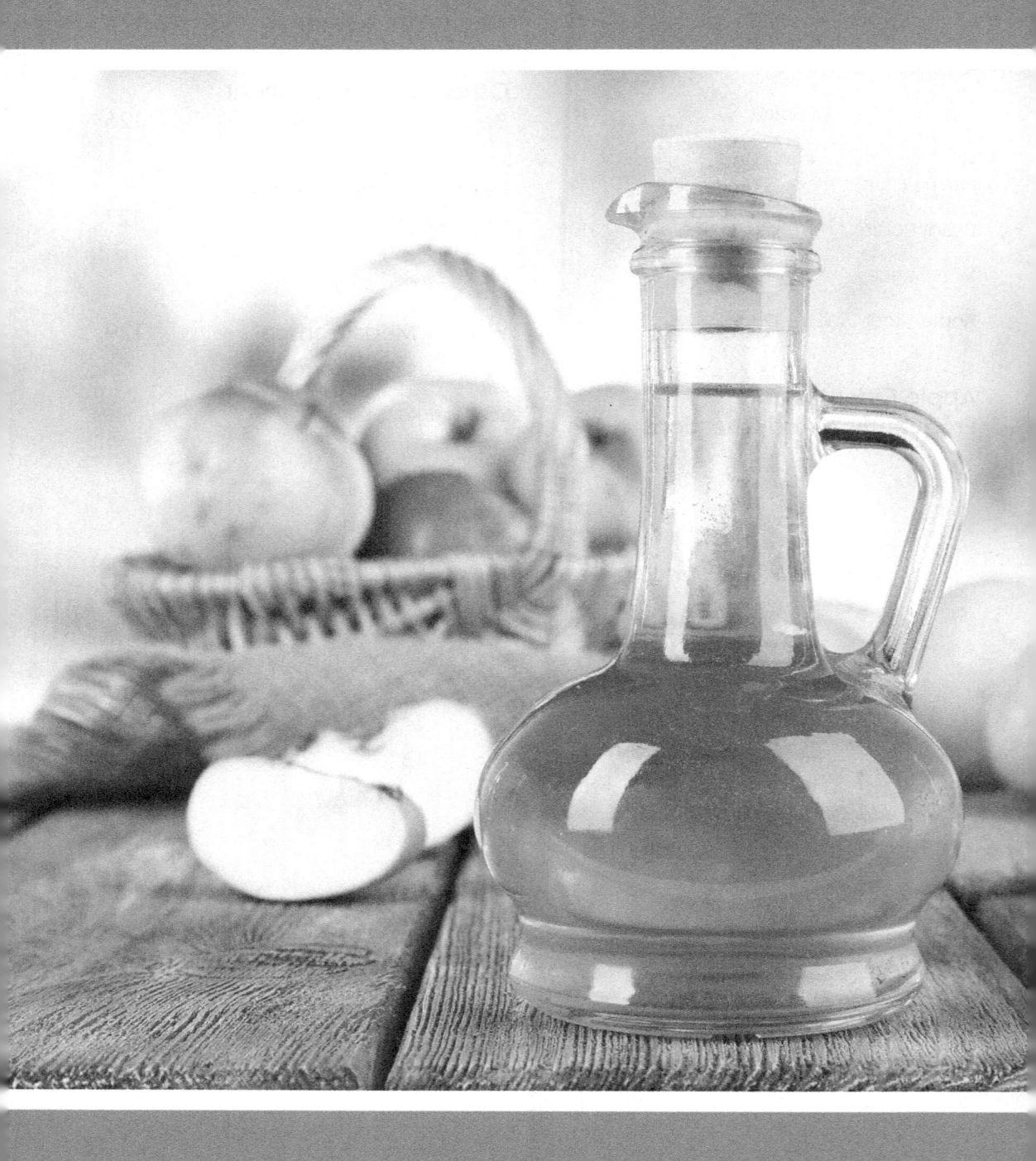

INTRODUCTION

Hi there

A very warm welcome to "The Apple Cider Vinegar Weight Loss Revolution," a weight loss plan designed for anyone who wants to lose weight and stay fit and active, but doesn't want to spend hours in the gym each week or go on a starvation diet.

In this book, I delve into the fascinating world of apple cider vinegar (ACV) and its potential role in weight loss and maintaining a healthy weight.

ACV has been gaining popularity as a natural remedy for weight loss and overall well-being for several years. Its unique composition – which includes beneficial enzymes, vitamins, and acetic acid - has intrigued health enthusiasts and researchers alike. However, amidst the buzz surrounding ACV, it is essential to separate fact from fiction and explore the scientific evidence behind its touted benefits.

In these pages, you will discover the truth about ACV and its potential as a weight loss aid. I aim to provide you with a comprehensive fat loss plan, backed by scientific research, expert insights, and practical tips, enabling you to make informed decisions about incorporating ACV into your own weight loss journey.

Throughout this book, I address crucial questions such as: How does ACV influence our metabolism? Can it truly help curb appetite and reduce calorie intake? What is the optimal way to consume ACV for weight loss? I also explore the potential benefits and risks associated with ACV, helping you understand its role as part of a holistic approach to weight management.

However, it is important to emphasize that there is no magical solution or quick fix for weight loss. This book encourages a balanced and evidence-based approach to health, with ACV serving as a potential tool to support your weight loss goals. I advocate a comprehensive lifestyle approach that includes a healthy diet, regular exercise, daily use of apple cider vinegar and a positive mindset.

Whether you are curious about ACV's weight loss benefits, looking to enhance your existing weight management routine, or simply seeking knowledge about this natural remedy, "The Apple Cider Vinegar Weight Loss Revolution" aims to be your trusted companion. I hope to provide you with the knowledge, strategies, and inspiration to embark on a sustainable weight loss journey with ACV as a potential ally.

Join me as I unravel the science, dispel myths, and guide you towards incorporating ACV into your everyday life in a safe and effective manner. Together, let's unlock the power of apple cider vinegar for sustainable weight loss and embrace a healthier, happier you.

I wish you the very best of luck and hope you enjoy every success with your weight loss journey.

To your health and fitness,

Jago Holmes CPT

WHAT IS APPLE CIDER VINEGAR?

> Apple cider vinegar has been used for centuries. It traces its roots back to ancient Babylon, around 5000 BC, where it was used as a tonic and a condiment.

Apple cider vinegar (or ACV as it is often referred to) is a type of vinegar made from fermented apple juice.

The use of apple cider vinegar dates back thousands of years and throughout history, man has been using vinegar for a range of purposes. We have been adding it to food for flavor, drinking it for its health-giving properties and using it to cleanse the body and the home for countless years.

The origins of vinegar production can be traced back to ancient civilisations, including the Babylonians, Egyptians, and Romans. These cultures used various fruits including apples - to create vinegar for use in cooking and medicine.

The Greek physician Hippocrates, often referred to as the "father of medicine," is said to have prescribed apple cider vinegar (mixed with honey) to fight illness and disease as early as 400BC and archaeologists have even discovered apple cider vinegar in Egyptian urns dating to around 3000BC!

During the Middle Ages, vinegar gained popularity as a versatile ingredient for cooking, food preservation, and hygiene. It was commonly used for pickling vegetables and other foods to increase the length of time they could be stored instead of having to be eaten straight away. Vinegar was also used as a condiment, and natural disinfectant.

As European settlers arrived in America, they brought the tradition of making vinegar with them. Apple orchards flourished in the New World, and apple cider vinegar became a common product of the harvests.

Throughout history, apple cider vinegar has been used in traditional folk medicine practices around the world. It was believed to have various health benefits, including aiding digestion, promoting weight loss, and treating ailments including sore throats and skin conditions.

In more recent times, apple cider vinegar has experienced a resurgence in popularity. It has gained attention as a natural remedy for weight loss, improving digestion, blood sugar control, and much more. This increased interest has led to scientific research exploring its properties and potential applications, which we will look into a little later in this book.

Today, apple cider vinegar is widely available in supermarkets, health food outlets, and online stores. It is used in a variety of culinary recipes, homemade remedies, and natural cleaning solutions.

How is Apple Cider Vinegar Produced?

Apple cider vinegar is basically created by the fermentation of apple cider or apple must (apple wine). The process is usually speeded up in mass production to make it quicker and easier to produce.

Here are the 3 main stages in the commercial production of this wonderful product, they are...

1. **Crushing and Pressing**: In this initial process apples are first washed and crushed to create apple pomace, which is a mixture of apple flesh, skin, and seeds. The pomace is then pressed to extract the liquid known as apple juice. This juice serves as the base for apple cider vinegar.

2. **Alcoholic Fermentation:** Next, yeast is added to the apple juice if a faster process is desired, otherwise yeast which naturally occurs on the skin of the apples is allowed to kick-start the fermentation of the apple juice on its own which turns the sugars present in the juice into alcohol, through a process called *alcoholic fermentation*. This step is similar to the fermentation that occurs during the production of most alcoholic drinks.

3. **Acetic Acid Fermentation:** During this final stage, the apple cider undergoes a transformation as it turns into vinegar. The alcohol produced from the fermentation is converted into acetic acid by bacteria. These bacteria convert the alcohol into acetic acid through a process known as *acetic acid fermentation*. This bacteria-driven process gives vinegar its characteristically sour taste. The fermentation process usually takes several weeks to many months, depending on various factors including temperature, oxygen exposure, the method used and the desired acidity level.

At this stage, there are a number of possible options, as it can be filtered, unfiltered or pasteurised or unpasteurised.

Some producers choose to leave the vinegar unfiltered and unpasteurised, which results in the presence of the "mother."

What is Apple Cider Mother?

Apple cider "mother" refers to a cloudy, stringy substance that appears in some unfiltered and unpasteurised varieties. It is often described as a cobweb-like formation or sediment that settles at the bottom of the fermentation casks.

It is composed of beneficial bacteria, enzymes, and proteins. It naturally forms during the fermentation process of apple cider vinegar. When apples are fermented into cider and then into vinegar, acetic acid

> One of the unique features of apple cider vinegar is the "mother." The mother is a cloudy substance made up of beneficial bacteria and enzymes that form during the fermentation process. It is often regarded as a sign of high-quality vinegar and contains many health-promoting properties.

bacteria convert the alcohol into acetic acid as we discussed earlier and it is when this process occurs, that the mother can develop and float in the vinegar.

It's important to note that while it is often associated with higher-quality apple cider vinegar and potential health benefits, scientific research on its specific effects is limited. Also, the exact composition and properties of the mother can vary between different brands and batches of apple cider vinegar.

Filtered and pasteurised apple cider vinegar is clear and does not contain the mother. It is worth mentioning that both filtered and unfiltered apple cider vinegar can be used in various culinary and household applications, but it is the unfiltered version with the mother that we are discussing here and is the one preferred by most people for its potential health benefits.

If you want to buy apple cider vinegar with the mother, be sure to choose unfiltered, and unpasteurised apple cider vinegar. If you're seeking the potential benefits associated with the mother and its components, then always carefully check the label or product description to ensure it contains the mother.

The presence of the mother is considered a good thing as it is believed to have additional health benefits, one of these is that it contains probiotics, which are beneficial bacteria that support our gut health.

What Are Probiotics?

Probiotics are live microorganisms, commonly referred to as "*good bacteria*," that provide health benefits when consumed in adequate amounts. These microorganisms are similar to the beneficial bacteria that naturally reside in our digestive tract.

Probiotics can be found in many food sources and dietary supplements other than ACV. They are most commonly associated with promoting digestive health, but research has also shown potential benefits for other aspects of health, such as immune function, and good skin health.

The most common types of probiotics belong to the groups *Lactobacillus* and *Bifidobacterium*, although there are many different strains within these groups. Each strain has its own unique properties and potential health benefits.

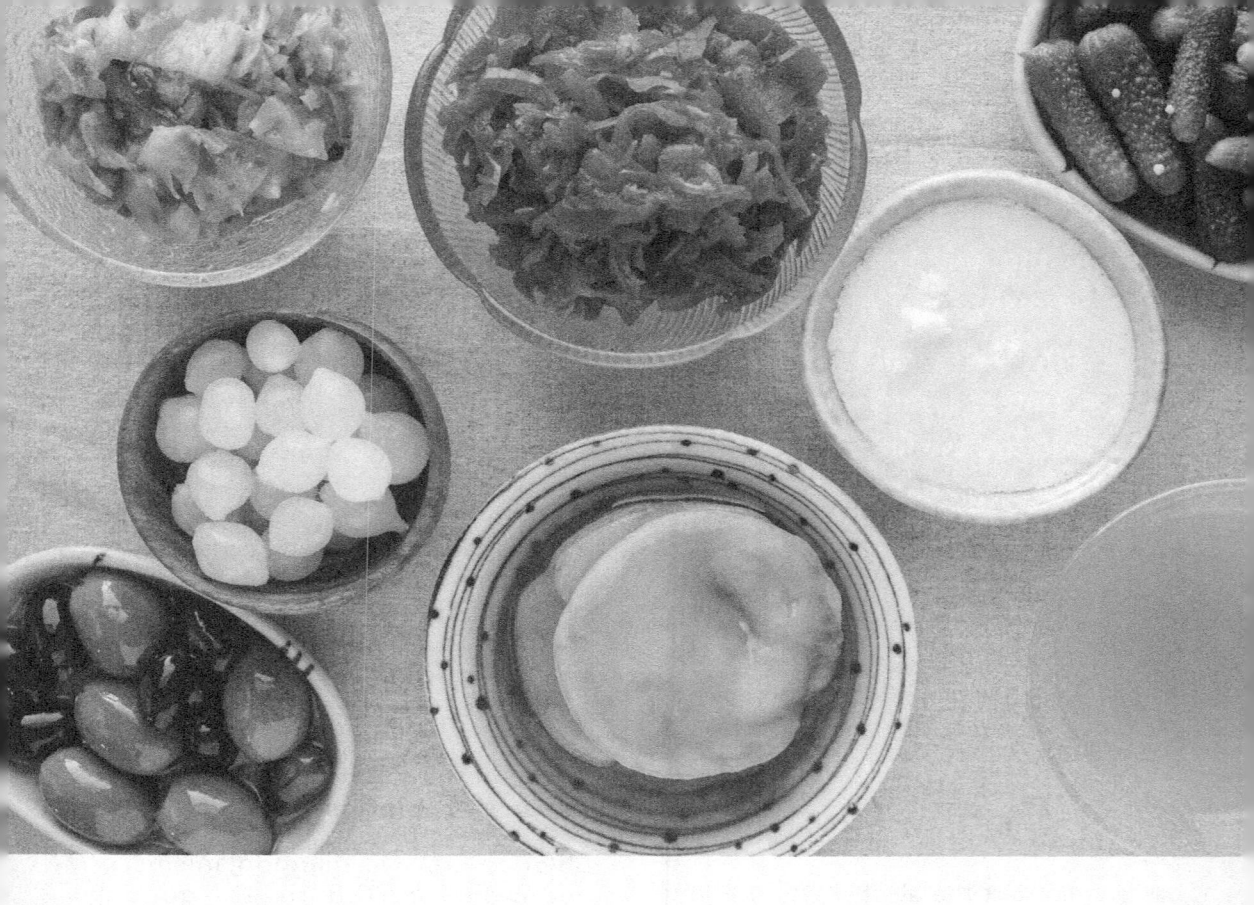

Why Are Probiotics Good for Us?

There are several reasons why it is a good idea to supplement your diet with probiotics...

Probiotics can...

- Help maintain a healthy balance of bacteria in the digestive system. They may assist in the breakdown of food, nutrient absorption, and the production of certain vitamins.

- Play an important role in supporting immune function. They may help regulate the immune response and promote a healthier gut barrier, which can contribute to overall immune system health.

- Help restore and maintain a healthy balance of bacteria in the gut microbiota, which is the complex community of microorganisms in our digestive system. Disruptions in this balance have been linked to various health issues.

- Improve mental health - Some studies suggest that certain probiotics may even have a positive impact on mental health conditions, such as anxiety, depression, and stress.

- Prevent or reduce diarrhoea associated with antibiotic use. Probiotics, especially certain strains of *Lactobacillus* and *Saccharomyces boulardii*, have been shown to help.

- Improve certain skin conditions, including acne, eczema, and rosacea.

You don't necessarily need to take a probiotic supplement to get these benefits as they occur naturally in many foods and drinks including (foods like) yogurt, kefir, sauerkraut, kimchi, and certain types of pickles. They are also available in the form of dietary supplements, including capsules, tablets, powders, and liquids.

While probiotics are generally considered safe and of benefit to most healthy people, anyone with a compromised immune system or serious health condition should consult a healthcare professional before use. Also, the effects of probiotics can vary from person to person, so it may take some trial and error to find the most suitable probiotic product for your needs, but ACV is a very good start.

Before we move on to look at the many benefits of ACV and how it can be used- particularly for weight loss - let's take a quick look at how you can make this amazing product for yourself in your own home, making it purer, cheaper, and more natural. Instead of adding bacteria, yeast etc., you can simply allow nature to run its course!

Making your own Apple Cider Vinegar

Making your own ACV is an ideal way to save money on expensive packaged versions and it is environmentally friendly as you aren't relying on ingredients being shipped over large distances, the damaging emissions from an industrial process or the use of disposable packaging.

However, the most important benefit of making your own ACV must be the fact that you have control over what is going into it; you can choose your apples, select your ingredients, and monitor the process all the way so you know exactly what you're getting. It is also a great way to use up a glut of apples if you grow your own or can buy a lot of them in bulk at a good price.

If you are interested in making your own ACV, the following instructions make it easy for you to create whole apple cider vinegar in your own home using the things you already have.

There is no need to use yeast with this method, so it will take longer - but it's well worth it. The only difficult part of the process is having the patience to wait until the ACV is ready for use!

WHOLE APPLE CIDER VINEGAR RECIPE

This is a simple method for making your own apple cider vinegar using whole apples, but you need to be patient as the fermentation process can take many months.

INGREDIENTS

- A large jar or ceramic crock (alternatively a big bowl will work)
- A piece of cheesecloth or cotton rag big enough to cover the top of the jar or bowl (twice) in a double layer
- Apples (preferably organic and washed well)
- Water
- Rubber band or string
- A dark and warm location to store the apple cider vinegar

METHOD

1. Wash the apples thoroughly to remove any dirt or residue. You can use any single variety of apples or a combination of different types. If possible, choose organic apples, as they won't have any traces of chemicals on the skin.

2. Remove the apple cores and chop the apples into quarters or thin slices. You don't need to peel the apples as this recipe is for whole apple cider vinegar, so we include the skins because they contain beneficial microorganisms.

3. Place the apples on a tray and allow them to turn brown in the air – this is the beginning of the process. It should take a few hours, maybe half a day for the apples to brown.

4. When the apples have browned, place them in the jar or bowl and cover them with water. Use mineral water or filtered tap water for this. If you want to speed up the process, you can add a tablespoon or two of sugar to help kick-start the fermentation process - although this is not necessary, purely optional.

5. Cover the bowl with the piece of cheesecloth – it is important you use cheesecloth as it allows air to circulate but stops anything (unwanted) falling into the bowl. We don't want an airtight cover as oxygen has to pass through the cover. Then secure the cheesecloth with a rubber band or string to keep out insects and dust.

6. Find a warm, dark cupboard with a temperature between 60 - 80°F (15-27°C) and place the covered bowl inside. Stir the mixture every few days to ensure proper oxygenation.

7. Allow the mixture to ferment for about 3- 4 weeks. Over time, there should be a layer of scum forming on top of the liquid. This is known as the "mother" of vinegar which indicates that fermentation is occurring, and (it)is a good sign!

8. Once the fermentation period is complete and the vinegar has reached your desired taste, strain out the solids using a fine-mesh sieve or cheesecloth. The liquid that remains is your homemade apple cider vinegar- with mother. You can discard the solids or use them in compost.

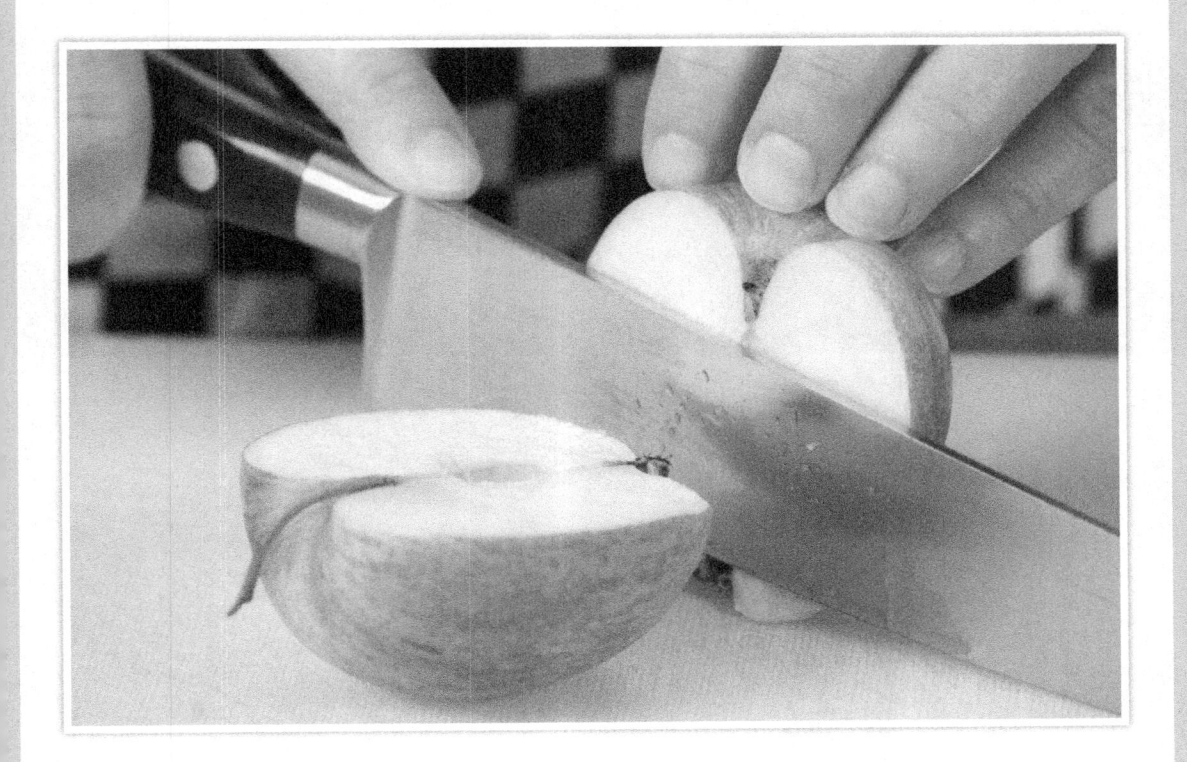

9. Aging (optional) - For a more robust flavor, you can choose to age the apple cider vinegar for a few more weeks in a cool, dark place before using it. This step is optional but can enhance the taste.
10. Finally transfer the vinegar to clean and sterilized glass bottles or jars, ensuring they are tightly sealed.

NOTE

During the fermentation process, it's normal for some sediment to settle at the bottom of the container. This is also a sign of natural fermentation.

Remember to always sterilize your equipment before use and maintain cleanliness throughout the process to prevent the growth of any harmful bacteria.

And there you have it; your own, homemade apple cider vinegar, ready for use.

Read on to find out how you can make the best use of your vinegar and the difference it could make to your life.

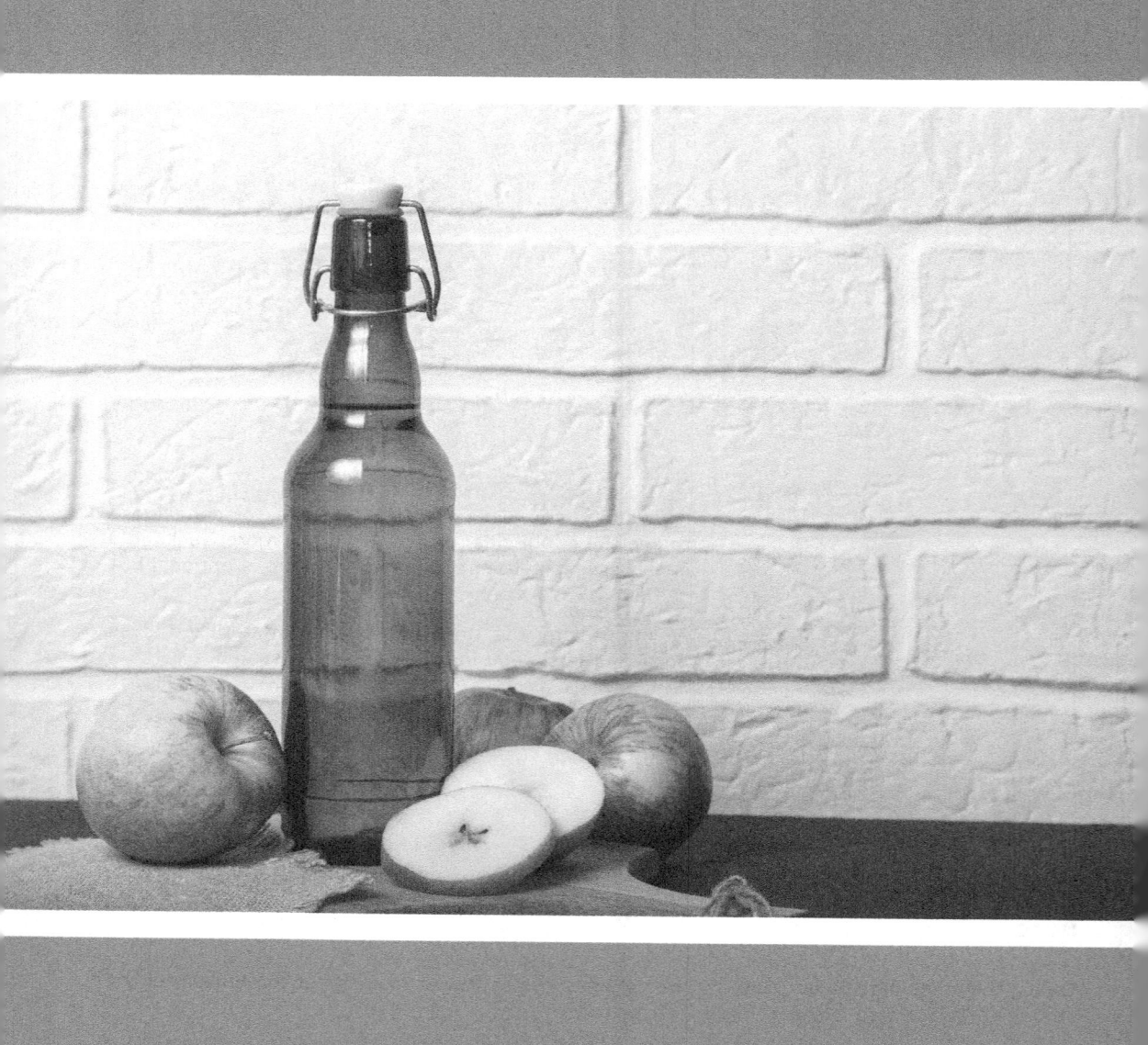

THE MANY HEALTH BENEFITS OF APPLE CIDER VINEGAR

Apple cider vinegar is known for its various health benefits. It has been linked to improved digestion, weight management, blood sugar control, and even potential antibacterial and antifungal properties.

ACV offers a wide range of health benefits and one of the most publicized and well-known of these is its reputation as a weight-loss aid. But before we move on to look at how apple cider vinegar can be used to boost weight loss, let's look at its considerable nutritional value and the other health benefits it can offer.

The Nutritional Value of Apple Cider Vinegar

Many people are surprised to learn just how much nutritional value ACV has. Many of us are so accustomed to thinking of vinegar as something we add to foods to enhance their taste, using it for flavor or when preserving other foods. that it comes as quite a shock to think of it as a nutritious substance in its own right.

Really it should be prized for its exceptional nutritional content.

VITAMINS

Apple cider vinegar has been found to contain the following vitamins, each of which has a range of important functions within the human body...

Vitamin A – for good vision, skin health, red blood cell production and a strong immune system.

Vitamin B1, B2 and B6 – essential for growth, development, and a healthy nervous system, also good for the metabolism.

Beta-carotene (a pro-vitamin) – the body converts this into vitamin A, and it is also an antioxidant, important for heart health.

Vitamin C – for immunity against disease and illness, cell renewal and boosting skin health; one of the most versatile vitamins.

Vitamin E – for healthy skin, nails and hair as well as protecting the body from free radicals.

MINERALS

ACV has been found to contain the following minerals and trace elements (this list is not exhaustive, but it does highlight some of the important minerals and trace elements that ACV can provide) ...

Calcium – for strong bones and teeth.

Phosphorus – benefits many bodily functions including digestion and growth.

Potassium – essential for organ function, including heart and liver health.

Sodium – an electrolyte needed in small amounts for a range of functions.

Sulphur – can ease allergies and help keep skin healthy.

Magnesium – needed for hundreds of biochemical reactions, helps absorb vitamins.

Iron – essential for many reasons, including transporting oxygen through the blood.

Copper – anti-ageing, essential for growth and development.

Silicon – known for beauty-promoting properties; benefits hair, skin, eyes, and nails.

The health improvements that can be gained through using apple cider vinegar are many. Before we look at the types of illness and health problems that ACV can benefit, it is important to understand some of the fundamental reasons why ACV is so potent. There are two essential systems that ACV can influence, which are...

- The acid/alkaline balance of the body
- The salt/fluid balance of the body

What is the Acid/Alkaline Balance and Why is it Important?

The balance of acid and alkaline in the body is important. The PH level of the body has an impact on health and wellbeing so it's worth noting that most people in the west have an overly acidic system. It is thought that many illnesses are brought on by a system that is over-acidic... by regulating the body's acid/alkaline balance you can experience increased energy, strength, and better overall health.

Although it may seem counter-intuitive that ACV could create a more alkaline PH level in the body, it can be proven by testing the urine before and after taking ACV for a period of time. It is also thought to bring a system that is too alkaline (although this is less common) back to a healthy level.

The result... a healthier body, stronger immune system, and renewed vitality.

How to Test Your PH Balance

Testing the pH balance is easily done at home, it's a simple process that can be done using pH test strips specifically designed for this purpose. Here's how you can test the pH balance in urine:

1. Purchase pH Test Strips: Obtain pH test strips from a pharmacy or online retailer. Look for strips specifically designed for testing urine pH.

2. Collect a Urine Sample: Collect a fresh urine sample in a clean container. The first urine of the day is often recommended for more accurate results.

3. Prepare the Test Strip: Remove a pH test strip from the packaging. Take care not to touch the testing area with your fingers, as it may affect the accuracy of the results.

4. Dip the Test Strip: Dip the testing end of the strip into the urine sample for a few seconds, making sure that the test area is fully immersed in the urine.

5. Remove Excess Urine: Gently shake off any excess urine from the strip to avoid dilution or contamination of the results. Follow the specific instructions provided with the test strips, as some may have different recommendations.

6. Wait for the Result: Place the test strip on a clean, dry surface and wait for the designated time indicated on the packaging or instructions. This is usually a few seconds to a minute.

7. Compare the Colors: After the designated time has passed, compare the color change on the test strip with the provided color chart or pH scale. Each color corresponds to a different pH level.

8. Determine the pH Level: Match the color of the test strip to the closest color on the chart to determine the pH level of your urine. The pH scale typically ranges from acidic (low pH) to alkaline (high pH).

Remember, a normal pH level for urine can vary depending on factors such as diet, hydration, medications, and underlying health conditions. Typically, the normal range for urine pH is between 5.0 and 8.0, with a slightly acidic to neutral pH considered normal.

If you have concerns about your urine pH or suspect any underlying health issues, it's always best to consult with a healthcare professional for a thorough evaluation and interpretation of your test results.

What is the Electrolyte/Fluid Balance of the Body and Why is it So Important?

The balance of electrolytes and fluid in the human body is an important one to maintain. Few of us realize that the level of fluid or electrolytes that we have in our blood changes, but we can feel the difference.

When the level of electrolytes is too high, the kidneys work to reduce it. When the level of electrolytes is low, ACV can be used to reduce sodium levels by removing sodium from the body. When our fluid levels are low, we experience thirst and fatigue. Strenuous exercise can lead to loss of both fluids and electrolytes; this is why people reach for sports drinks which are designed to replenish both.

Hydrating with electrolytes and fluids together provides faster, more effective hydration and helps the fluids we take in become absorbed into the body more easily, rather than passed out in the urine. So where does apple cider vinegar come in?

Many athletes use a little ACV in water to replenish electrolyte levels and boost hydration as it gives a very fast dose of essential electrolytes and helps to balance the system.

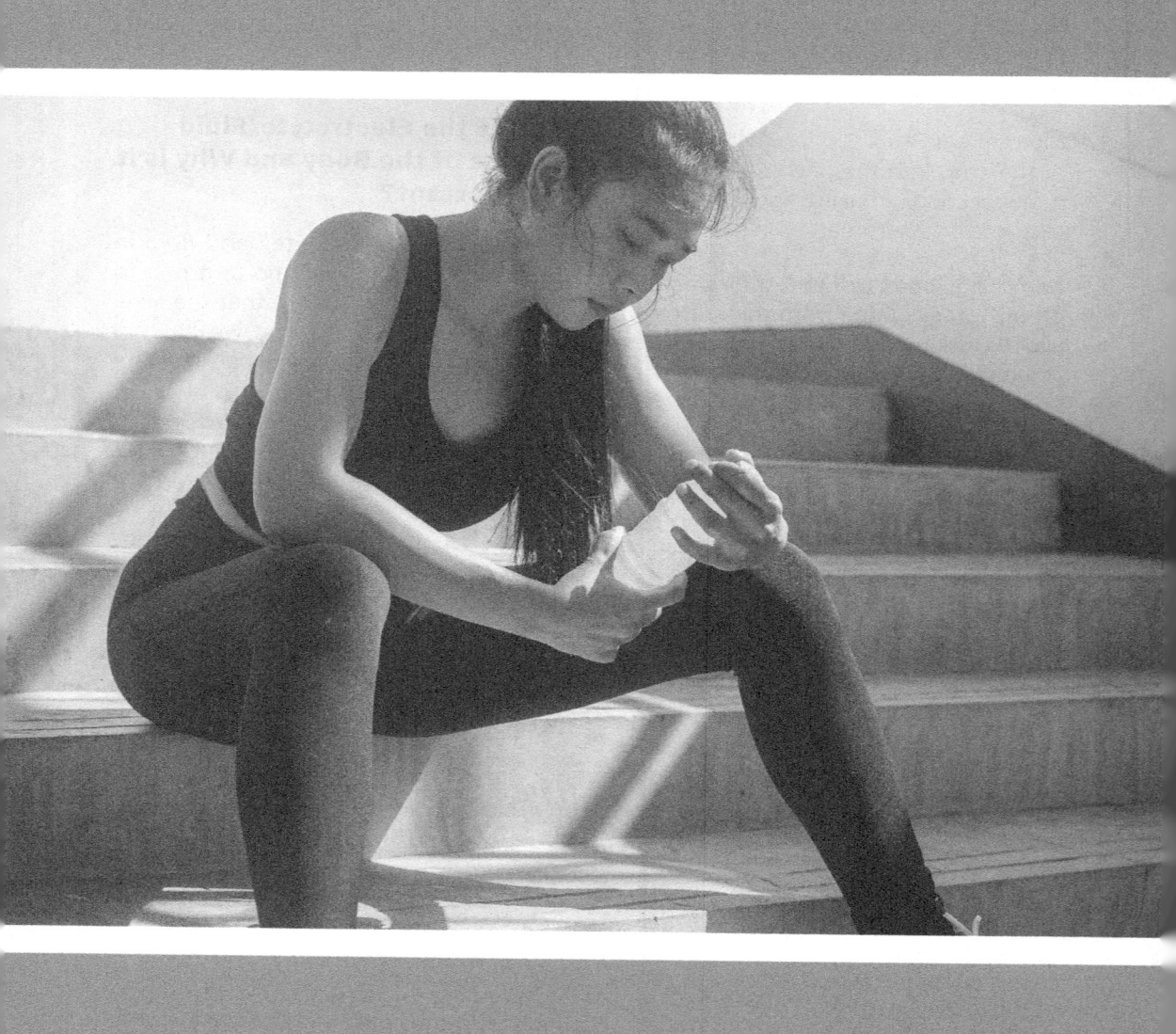

HEALTH PROBLEMS AND APPLE CIDER VINEGAR

> Despite its acidic nature, some people use apple cider vinegar as a natural teeth whitening remedy. The theory is that the acidic properties can help remove stains from the surface of teeth. However, it's important to exercise caution as prolonged or excessive use can erode tooth enamel, so it's best to consult with a dentist before attempting this method.

Apple cider vinegar has had reported benefits for people with all kinds of illnesses, diseases, and health complaints. The following are some of the most common problems that could be helped by ACV.

It is extremely important to discuss the pros and cons of taking any supplement or using different treatments for an illness with a medical professional who knows your history.

If you feel your doctor is skeptical, ask them to investigate it for you or at least have them agree that ACV won't do any harm (even if they aren't willing to admit that it may do a lot of good!)

High LDL (bad) Cholesterol

The water-soluble dietary fiber found in apple cider vinegar (specifically in the pectin) can help lower LDL cholesterol. LDL is the dangerous form of cholesterol, high levels of which can cause heart problems. As well as this, it is thought that the amino acids (with) in ACV could work to help eliminate oxidized LDL cholesterol which is particularly dangerous.

LDL Cholesterol is a scourge of the modern age and yet it can be reduced by making various dietary and lifestyle changes. Apple cider vinegar can help reduce cholesterol levels safely and quickly, making it a real benefit for those at risk of high cholesterol levels or heart disease.

Arthritis

Apple cider vinegar has been shown to reduce pain in those suffering from arthritis; this is likely down to its action on eliminating toxins that build up in the body.

Circulatory Problems

Apple cider vinegar is thought to stimulate the circulation and at the same time can lower blood pressure… a double benefit.

Water Retention

Apple cider vinegar is high in potassium which can help reduce fluid retention. This can help the appearance, reducing swelling and discomfort.

Cancer

Apple cider vinegar won't fight against cancer, but it can fight the free radicals that experts increasingly believe to be behind some cancers. It can also be hugely beneficial in maintaining better health during treatment and recovery.

Ulcers

Apple cider vinegar is often used to treat stomach ulcers; it may come as a surprise, but many sufferers have found relief as the ACV balances the acid in the gastrointestinal tract.

Digestive Problems

By stimulating the digestive system, ACV is believed to help break down food in the stomach more efficiently, while regulating the system and helping to normalize the body's acid/alkaline balance – all this means a more efficient, more comfortable digestive system.

Those who suffer from constipation or diarrhea can also benefit from the balancing properties of apple cider vinegar.

Liver Problems

Apple cider vinegar is frequently used to cleanse the liver. This enables it to function more effectively and efficiently, allowing it to carry on with the important job of getting rid of waste products.

Vision

There are many people who swear by taking ACV in water to improve problems with vision and maintain eye health. Others use a very weak solution of ACV in tepid water to swab the eyes to get rid of conjunctivitis and styes. There is a lot of anecdotal evidence that this works - most likely down to the cleansing and balancing effect ACV has on the whole body.

COMMON DAY TO DAY AILMENTS THAT ACV CAN HELP

> Unlike many other food products, apple cider vinegar has an incredibly long shelf life. Due to its high acidity, it has natural preservative properties, which means it can last indefinitely without spoiling.

As well as long term health problems and diseases, apple cider vinegar can be used to treat common day to day ailments that commonly occur. These may not be life-threatening or cause much pain, but anything that affects your quality of life can stop you from enjoying true good health.

Using a natural remedy like ACV allows you to save money, time and effort and can give you better results than many of the commercially available preparations...

Candida

This systemic problem can be treated by taking ACV in water or in herbal tea or by adding a cup of ACV to a relaxing bath; fighting the internal and external symptoms to rid the body of an overgrowth of candida which can cause a range of issues from fatigue to sugar cravings.

Warts

You can remove a wart using apple cider vinegar; it works quickly and leaves no scar, and it is safer and cheaper than some chemical preparations you can buy. Simply place a cotton ball dipped in the ACV onto the wart and cover with a bandage and leave overnight, repeat for a few days until the wart changes color (turns brown or black) after which time the wart should fall off.

Nasal Congestion

Taking a teaspoon of ACV in a small glass of warm water has been known to help sinus and nasal congestion helping to relieve stuffy noses and ease cold symptoms.

> Apple cider vinegar can be used as a natural and eco-friendly household cleaner. Its acidic nature makes it effective at removing stains, odors, and bacteria. It can be used to clean surfaces, appliances, and even as a natural fabric softener.

Sore Throat

Simply gargle with a solution of 1 part ACV to 2 parts tepid water. Repeat 3 times a day for relief from sore throats.

Aches, pains, and joint stiffness

In the same way that apple cider vinegar can ease the symptoms of arthritis, it can also ease other aches and pains caused by inflammation. Take in the usual way in water and see if you feel a difference.

Allergies

ACV has been found to ease the symptoms of allergies; from pet allergies to hay-fever. It appears to lower the body's response to allergens so you can experience relief from itching, runny nose and eye and skin reactions.

Sunburn

It may not seem like the most soothing of balms, but apple cider vinegar can bring real relief to sunburnt skin. Simply dip a flannel or soft towel in a bowl of water with a few tablespoons of ACV added and wrap the affected area. Leave for 30 minute and refresh and reapply for long lasting relief from discomfort and burning. PLEASE NOTE: Do NOT add neat apple cider vinegar to the affected area.

Acne

ACV can ease the inflammation of acne and help to safely dry spots and prevent them spreading. Apply a moderate solution (1 part ACV to 1 part water) to the affected area and then rinse well, dry well and be careful not to let the skin get too dry.

Dandruff

An itchy flaky scalp can be incredibly frustrating (and embarrassing). Rinsing the hair with a solution of 1:1 water/ACV can help clear dandruff and leave your hair squeaky clean, just rinse thoroughly with warm water afterwards.

Some of the above is supported only by anecdotal evidence and there are few studies to back up the claims other than historical evidence of its use.

HOW TO CHOOSE APPLE CIDER VINEGAR

> While apple cider vinegar should not be applied directly to sunburned skin, adding a cup of apple cider vinegar to a cool bath can provide relief. The vinegar's natural properties can help balance the skin's pH level and potentially soothe sunburned skin.

When choosing a brand of apple cider vinegar, consider the following factors to make an informed decision:

1. Organic and raw: Look for ACV that is labelled as "organic" to ensure it is made from organically grown apples without the use of synthetic pesticides or fertilizers. Additionally, opt for ACV that is labelled as "raw" or "unfiltered." Raw ACV is minimally processed and retains the "mother," which is a cloudy substance containing beneficial enzymes and bacteria.

2. Quality and purity: Choose a reputable brand that prioritizes quality control and maintains high standards in production. Look for ACV that is made from pure apple juice without additives, preservatives, or artificial colors.

3. Acidity level: ACV typically has an acidity level of 5% acetic acid. Ensure that the brand you choose maintains this standard acidity level, as it is necessary for its potential health benefits.

4. Transparency and certifications: Look for brands that provide transparency about their sourcing and production methods. Certifications such as USDA Organic or Non-GMO Project Verified can offer additional assurance of quality and adherence to specific standards.

5. Packaging: ACV is commonly available in glass bottles or plastic containers. Glass bottles can help preserve the quality of ACV and prevent potential leaching from plastic. However, if you opt for plastic containers, ensure they are made of food-grade materials and are BPA-free.

6. Reviews and recommendations: Read reviews and seek recommendations from trusted sources, friends, or family members who have experience with different brands of ACV. Their insights can provide valuable information about the taste, quality, and effectiveness of various brands.

7. Price: Consider your budget, but keep in mind that cheaper options may compromise on quality or may not offer the desired benefits. Balance cost with quality to find a brand that suits your needs.

Ultimately, personal preference and individual responses may vary, so it may be worthwhile to try different brands and see which one works best for you.

There are organic versions, and some that are preservative free; make sure you check the product details out before you make your purchase, the fewer added ingredients, the better.

Look for cloudy ACV as this is a clue that it contains the "mother" which holds much of the nutritional value of the vinegar.

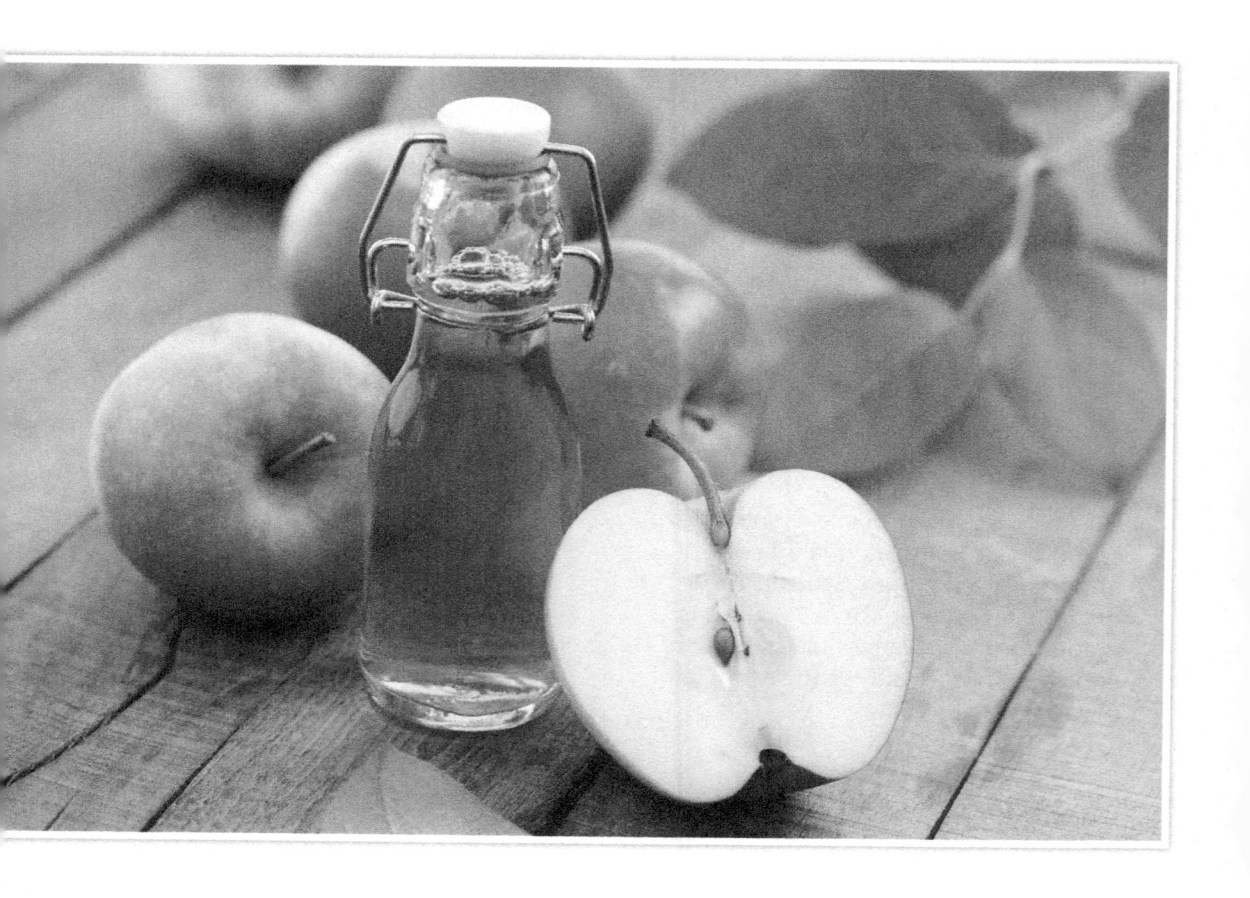

APPLE CIDER VINEGAR FOR WEIGHT LOSS

The reputation of ACV for boosting and maintaining weight loss is very strong and this is the focus of the rest of this book.

Many people, all over the world, are using apple cider vinegar to kick-start, boost and maintain a healthy weight loss program. It has been used for hundreds of years to help people slim down and embrace a fitter, healthier body.

How Does it Work?

So, just how does ACV help you lose weight?

Well, there are several factors involved. Once we've examined why and how it works, we will look at practical ways that you can make it work in your own life; looking at how to take ACV for weight loss and then moving onto other ways you can add it to your diet in the next chapter which also discuss how to make meals which include ACV.

Let's start with the 6 main factors that can help with weight loss...

1. Increased feelings of fullness: Some studies suggest that consuming ACV before meals may help increase satiety and reduce calorie intake. The acetic acid in ACV has been theorised to slow down the rate at which food leaves the stomach, leading to a longer lasting feeling of fullness. As a result, individuals may consume fewer calories overall.

2. Reduced appetite and cravings: ACV may help suppress appetite and cravings, potentially leading to reduced calorie consumption. However, the mechanisms behind this effect are not well understood, and more research is needed to support these claims.

3. Improved blood sugar control: ACV can play a role in regulating blood sugar levels, meaning you feel fuller for longer as there is less of a spike in your blood sugar after eating, which means less of a drop later. It is this drop in blood sugar levels that makes us crave sugary food. Think about that mid-afternoon slump a few hours after eating lunch when you're tempted to reach for a snack to perk you up and keep you going - that's your blood sugar levels dropping.

   High blood sugar levels can contribute to weight gain and difficulties in losing weight. Some studies have shown that consuming ACV with a high-carbohydrate meal can help lower post-meal blood sugar spikes. By stabilising blood sugar levels, ACV may reduce cravings and normalize the appetite by keeping the blood sugar level more stable and balanced. ACV can also slow down the speed at which the body digests starch, so you feel fuller for longer.

4. Reduces fat acumination: ACV may also help reduce fat accumulation because Acetic acid, found in apple cider vinegar, can make the body store fewer fatty deposits. This can be particularly useful in reducing harmful fatty deposits around the organs which can be especially bad for our health.

5. Water Retention: Many people suffer from water retention. While this is not fat, it certainly looks like fat, and it can add anything from an extra few ounces to pounds of extra weight at certain times.

   Many women find that they retain water at certain times in their menstrual cycles while others find that some medications they take- including birth

> Its medicinal properties have been recognized for centuries, and it was commonly used by ancient civilizations, including the Egyptians and Romans.

control pills- may make them retain water. The result is a bloated look and a sluggish feeling. This in turn makes it more difficult (and much less appealing) to exercise.

The good news is that there is a lot of anecdotal evidence that apple cider vinegar can help with water retention – so many people taking ACV experience a noticeable difference quite quickly because they are retaining less fluid. Combined with drinking plenty of water and exercise, this loss of retained fluid can boost weight loss as the body sheds toxins as well as fluid. The reason for this is the action of the ACV on the levels of potassium in the body; more potassium helps to flush sodium out of the body, and this in turn affects the salt/fluid balance.

6. Apple Cider Vinegar and Metabolism: ACV is believed to have a positive effect on the metabolic rate, speeding it up so we burn more calories in a shorter amount of time. The reason for this is again down to the acetic acid that ACV contains.

Many people claim that taking ACV has made their metabolism faster and more efficient and experts are continually examining these claims to try to identify exactly why this is happening. There are many theories, but the most likely one lies in the action of acetic acid on foods during digestion.

Acetic acid can help the body absorb the iron found in foods and this in turn boosts the amount of oxygen used, thus increasing the metabolic rate.

Ok, this is all well and good, but what about the science?

Well, there have been a number of scientific studies that have explored the benefits of ACV on weight loss, the most notable are as follows...

A study published in the Journal of Functional Foods (2018) examined the effects of ACV on postprandial (after-meal) blood glucose and satiety in healthy individuals. The researchers found that ACV consumption with a carbohydrate-rich meal led to lower blood sugar and insulin levels compared to a control group.

A small study published in the European Journal of Clinical Nutrition (2005) investigated the impact of vinegar on feelings of satiety (fullness). The researchers found that participants who consumed vinegar with a high-carbohydrate meal reported increased satiety compared to those who consumed a placebo with a high carbohydrate meal instead.

In a study on mice conducted by experts in 2009, it was discovered that as well as lowering LDL cholesterol (the bad cholesterol we should avoid), there was also a reduction in accumulated fat and liver lipids.

In another study published in the European Journal of Clinical Nutrition (2010) investigated the effects of vinegar supplementation on glucose and insulin responses in healthy subjects. The study found that ACV supplementation reduced postprandial glucose and insulin levels and increased feelings of satiety after a bread meal.

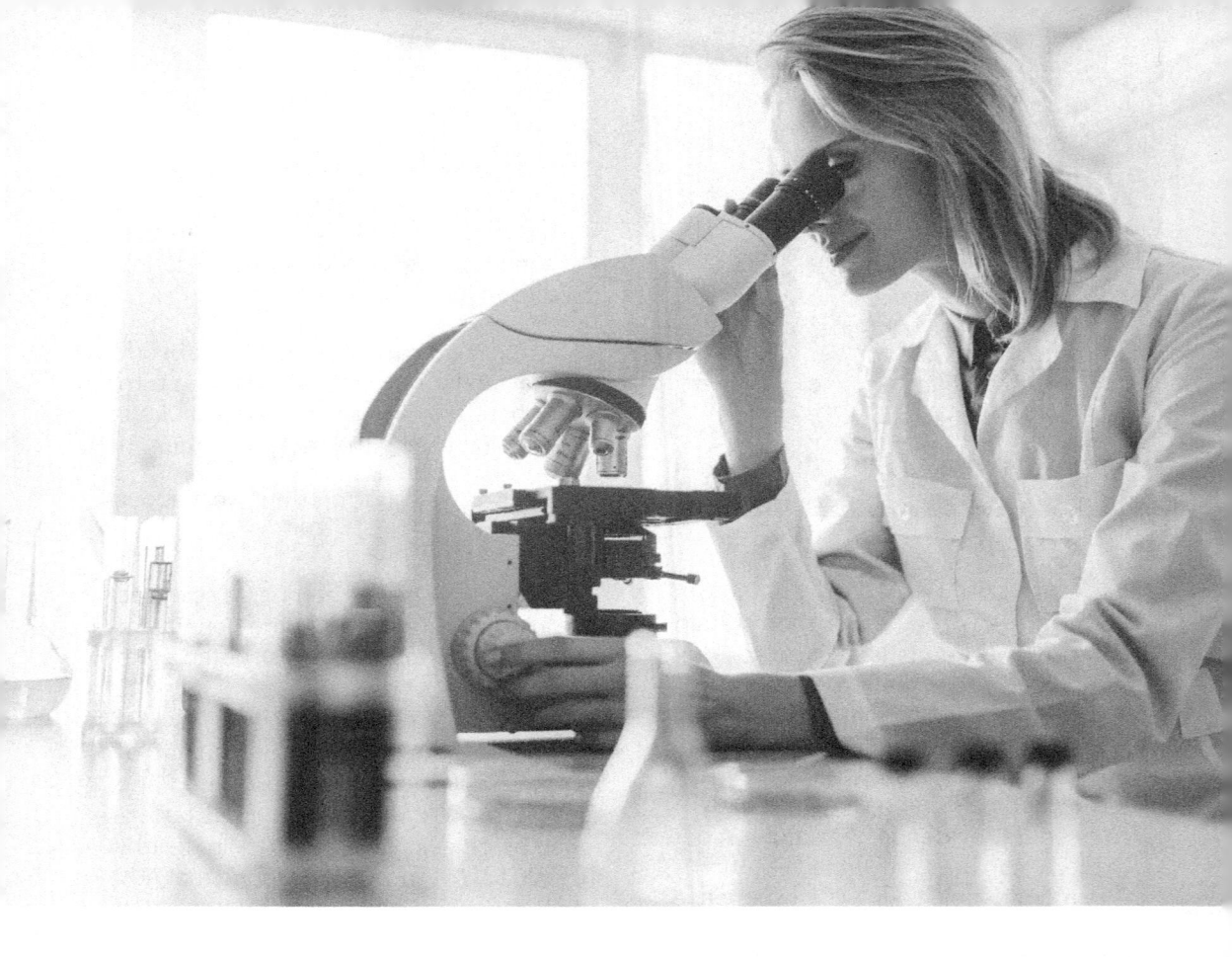

Another study testing the role of ACV as an appetite suppressant, was examined by experts in 2006 and reported in the Medscape Journal of Medicine. Their conclusion was - *"There is a direct relationship between increased acetic acid and satiety."* Elin Ostman, Lund University.

Finally, a study published in the Journal of Agricultural and Food Chemistry (2011) examined the anti-obesity effects of acetic acid - the main component of vinegar- on mice fed a high-fat diet. The results suggested that acetic acid might help regulate body weight and fat accumulation by altering gene expression related to fatty acid metabolism.

On his daytime TV show, Dr Mehmet Oz discussed the potential health benefits of apple cider vinegar and, more importantly, for its use in weight loss. He suggested that consuming ACV before meals may help reduce appetite and increase feelings of fullness. He also talked about how ACV could regulate blood sugar levels.

Also, Dr Oz mentioned that ACV might have potential digestive benefits. It is believed that the acetic acid in ACV could help improve digestion by increasing the production of stomach acid. However, scientific evidence to support these claims is currently limited.

Acetic Acid Benefits...

When consumed as part of apple cider vinegar (ACV), acetic acid - the main component of vinegar - can potentially have various effects on the body. Here are a few other ways acetic acid from apples may positively impact the body:

Appetite and satiety: As discussed above, acetic acid has been theorized to affect appetite and feelings of fullness. It may help increase satiety, potentially leading to reduced calorie intake. The exact mechanisms are not well understood, but it's believed that acetic acid may affect the central nervous system and appetite-regulating hormones.

Digestion and gut health: Acetic acid, like other types of vinegar, is known to possess antimicrobial properties that can help inhibit the growth of certain harmful bacteria.

Metabolism and fat storage: There is limited evidence to suggest that acetic acid may have an impact on metabolism and fat storage. Some studies conducted on animals and cells have indicated that acetic acid might influence genes and enzymes involved in fat metabolism. However, more research is needed to determine its effects on human metabolism and body fat regulation.

A Note on Patience

It should be noted that apple cider vinegar is not going to transform you overnight, but it will work if you stick to it, and the changes will be gradual. This is a healthy, natural way to change the way your body functions, but it isn't a quick fix that will land you right back at square one after a while either.

Apple cider vinegar is best used as a supplement to a healthy lifestyle. With a healthy diet, and increasing the amount of activity, exercise and strengthening you do, ACV will boost your efforts and help you to see better results. As the vinegar works to make you feel healthier and reduces any of the problems we have looked at in the previous chapter, you'll feel more in control of your body and more able to embrace a healthier lifestyle.

It is only natural that if apple cider vinegar means fewer aches and pains, or relief from arthritic complaints, you'll be more able and willing to exercise more. In the same way, relief from the discomfort of digestive problems will boost your energy and confidence levels.

The healthier you feel, the more energy you have, and all of this helps to contribute to the lifestyle changes you need to make in order to lose weight.

Apple cider vinegar provides you with a healthy, natural way to boost not just your weight loss, but your whole body. It is a holistic approach to weight loss and health that can truly make a difference to so many aspects of your life.

Boosting the Effects of Apple Cider Vinegar

As we have discussed, ACV purely on its own won't make the transformative impact on your body that you want. To see truly big changes, it's best to optimize the effects of using apple cider vinegar by making other simple lifestyle changes too.

We all know that making positive changes to your diet and increasing activity levels are the key to keeping calorie intake down and calorie burn up, but these are two easy ways to make a change to your health and wellbeing, boosting weight loss and increasing motivation.

ACV WEIGHT LOSS METHOD 1

There are many ways to use apple cider vinegar in a weight loss plan. In method 1 we focus on the simplest technique.

It's pretty straight forward – Before you eat any meal or snack throughout the day, you should have one of the following drinks - including before breakfast. (Don't forget this one as many people believe it is the most valuable time to take ACV when you wake, first thing in the morning before eating).

OPTION 1

Diluted with water: Mix 1 to 2 tablespoons of ACV with a glass of water (8-16 ounces) and drink it. It's important to dilute ACV with water because undiluted vinegar can be harsh on tooth enamel and the throat. Start with a lower amount of ACV and gradually increase it if desired.

OPTION 2

A comforting mug of ACV: Add 1 tablespoon of ACV to a mug and add 1 tablespoon of raw honey (Manuka honey is best as it has its own health-giving properties) and a slice of lemon, then pour on hot (but not boiling) water and sip as you would drink tea.

OPTION 3

ACV shot: Some people prefer taking a straight shot of ACV, followed by drinking water or rinsing the mouth to minimize contact with tooth enamel. This method is an acquired taste and allows for quick consumption - but can be strong and a little harsh tasting.

And that's it!!

Obviously to get the most benefit from using method one, you should increase your activity levels and eat a healthy, clean diet whenever possible – Or at the very least reduce your calorie intake, by limiting processed and junk foods where you can, but more on that in method 2, next.

If you try this for 7 days and lose weight, then you don't need to try either method 2 or 3, just keep going, but if this doesn't give you the results you were looking for, then you should move on to method 2 – The apple cider vinegar 'cleanse'

ACV WEIGHT LOSS METHOD 2

Method 2 is where we are going to go a little deeper into the use of apple cider vinegar and combine it with other wholesome foods to do a healthy, energy giving detox for a week.

An apple cider detox or "cleanse" is a type of detox or cleansing regime that involves the use of apple cider vinegar alongside eating and drinking other cleansing and pure, natural foods. It's a great way to cleanse or detoxify and improve overall health, flush toxins from the body, support digestion, boost metabolism, and aid in weight loss.

You should think of a detox for your body like a reboot is to a computer. As your PC updates the software and removes all the old files and programs that you don't need anymore – Similarly to the way a detox works to revitalise and nourish your body.

For our ACV cleanse you'll be doing 2 things...

Firstly, drinking a mixture of ACV and water with lemon juice, honey, and cayenne pepper, 3 times a day before meals for a week.

Secondly, eating a wide range of fresh, natural, wholesome healthy foods, with no processed or junk food or drinks at all.

Now I'll be honest, this won't be one of the easiest things you've ever tried, but if you do put the effort in and stick to the plan for the full 7 days without cheating, I promise you'll look and feel a lot better and have lost weight, guaranteed!!

The good thing about a detox, is that it's only strict for a short amount of time. After that, theoretically you should go back to eating a healthy balanced diet and exercising regularly to maintain the weight loss that you've achieved.

This detox is an ideal way to...

- Begin a new diet
- Start a lifestyle change
- Boost flagging energy levels
- Increase wellbeing
- Regain control when you have been over-indulging
- Get back on track when weight loss begins to slow down

Using apple cider vinegar to detoxify your body is an ideal starting point for weight loss and better health. This is not a brutal or dangerous detox program; it's a gentle and energizing cleanse so you can use it every few weeks without causing stress or damage to the body.

The success of this program lies with your dedication to being organized, buying fresh, raw produce in advance, and taking the ACV as described each day.

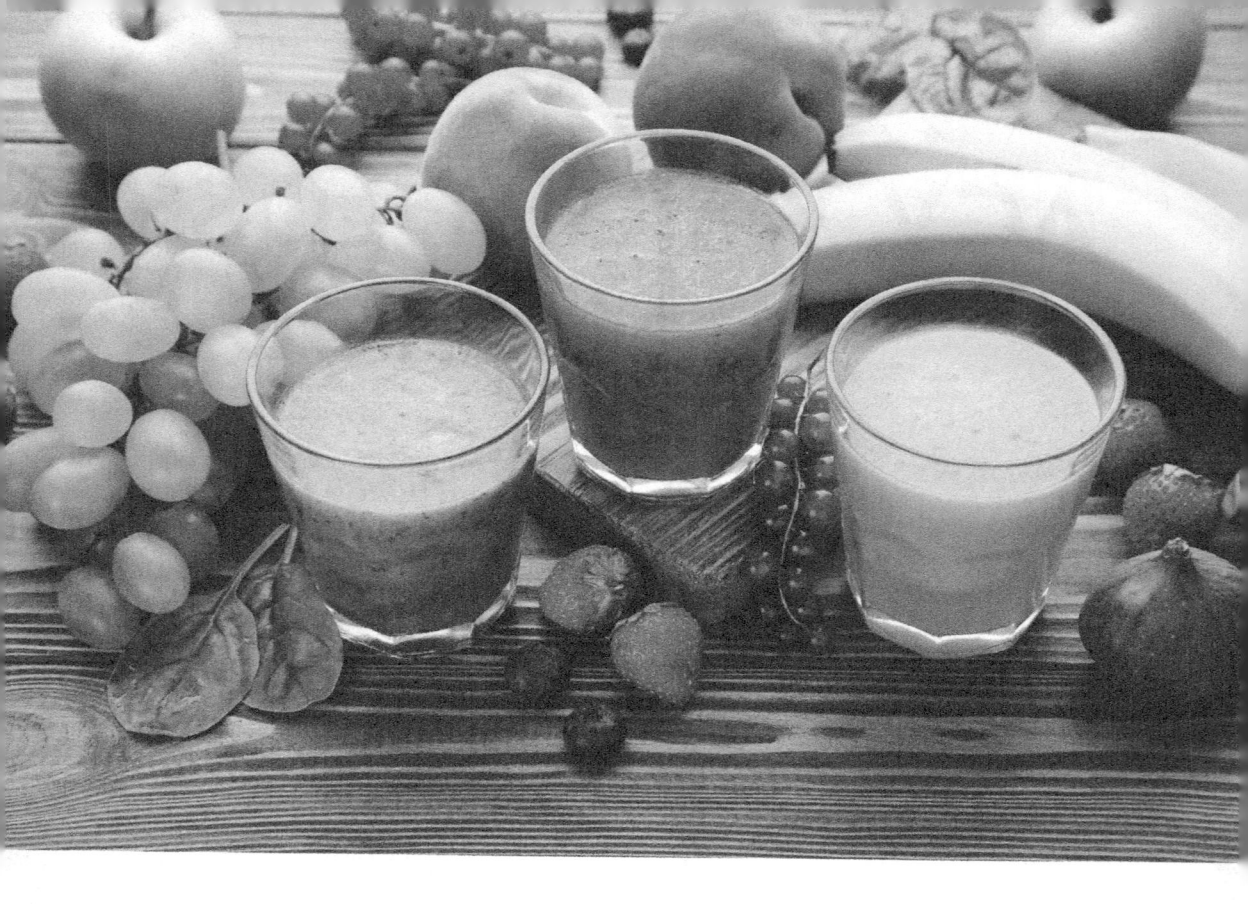

It's important to note that the effects of ACV on fasting will vary among individuals, and the scientific evidence regarding its impact on fasting is limited.

With that being said, let's get to the nitty, gritty - Here is what you need to do for the next 7 days...

How to Detox the Easy Way

Be organized; buy the fresh ingredients you need for your detox, plan ahead of time, so you're never tempted to skip your detox in favor of a quick fix.

ACV: take a tablespoon of apple cider vinegar in a glass of water before every meal and try to incorporate it in meals whenever possible.

Eat raw salads; fruit, and vegetables in their natural state; focus on organic raw ingredients and avoid all processed foods completely.

Avoid all processed grains, like bread, pastries, baked goods, and breakfast cereals.

Don't eat dairy; it's important for any good detox to avoid anything that contains dairy products.

Color: aim to eat the entire rainbow of colors in your diet plan every day.

Clean; stick to ACV for cleaning your home and body to reduce your exposure to chemicals and help eliminate toxins further. (Don't worry, there's a section on this later in the book)

Drink, drink, and drink; the more water you drink the better. Avoid caffeine, sugar, or artificially sweetened beverages and absolutely no alcohol. Aim to drink a total of 2 – 3 liters of water a day.

Exercise; make extra time for aerobic exercise like walking or cycling and gentle stretching exercises such as yoga or Pilates every day.

Relax; try to find gentle ways to relax, practice deep breathing and rest when you can to reduce stress.

Use extra virgin olive oil, and natural sea salt if you want to add a little more flavor to your foods or try adding minced garlic or ginger or thinly sliced fresh chili.

These are quite loose rules, so you've got a lot to think about before you start. Basically, anything grown in the ground or from trees is ok as long as it's in its natural state. So, a raw or cooked carrot would be fine, but as part of this detox we don't want you to make anything else to go with it - unless you're combining it with other raw foods to make your own soup or smoothie for example.

To give you an idea of what you should be eating, here's a sample detox day along with the recipes for the main meal it contains…

Before breakfast: ACV drink

Breakfast: Fresh fruit and berries and a handful of raw seeds or nuts of your choice (unsalted and not roasted)

Before lunch: ACV drink

Lunch: Baked sweet potato + steamed broccoli or carrots + piece of steamed fresh fish or oven baked free-range chicken breast

Before dinner: ACV drink

Dinner: Mixed leaf salad with apple cider vinegar dressing + piece of steamed fresh fish or oven baked free-range chicken or turkey breast.

Before bed: Herbal or fruit tea with ACV and honey

Here's how to make the drinks and dressing…

ACV DRINK

Mix one tablespoon of ACV with an 8-ounce glass of water, add a squeeze of lemon juice, a tablespoon of honey or natural maple syrup and a small pinch of cayenne pepper and drink it.

Apple cider vinegar is known for its pungent aroma, which happens to be irresistible to fruit flies. If you've ever had a fruit fly problem in your home, you may have encountered this fact firsthand. Placing a small dish of apple cider vinegar with a drop of dish soap can act as a trap, luring fruit flies in and effectively reducing their numbers.

APPLE CIDER VINEGAR, HONEY, AND MUSTARD DRESSING

A good honey-mustard dressing can work wonders for a salad and this one certainly does, warming and sweetening any collection of mixed leaves, from your basic salad ingredients to the more exotic concoctions. This works perfectly with an all-green salad but feel free to add whatever salad vegetables you want.

This dressing can be used for many salads if it is kept in a refrigerator in between uses.

INGREDIENTS

- ⅓ cup olive oil
- ⅓ cup apple cider vinegar
- 1 tbsp Dijon mustard
- 2 tbsp honey
- 3 tbsp fresh chives, finely chopped
- 1 clove garlic, finely minced
- 3 tbsp lemon juice
- Pinch salt

METHOD

1. In a large bowl, combine all ingredients well, reserving the olive oil.
2. Slowly mix the olive oil into the mixture, whisking very well to ensure a smooth result.
3. 3. Refrigerate for at least 30 minutes before serving.

If you feel hungry in between meals as you probably will do, snack on things like a handful of seeds, grapes, baby tomatoes or a few olives etc., but do so in moderation.

FRUIT OR HERBAL TEA WITH APPLE CIDER VINEGAR

Add your favorite fruit or herbal tea bag to a cup, pour over freshly boiled water and allow to sit for 2 or 3 minutes, then add 1 tbsp of ACV and 1 tsp pure honey or natural maple syrup, stir and enjoy.

You'll find plenty of healthy meals in the back of the book and whilst these recipes contain ACV and are great options for weight loss, not all will be suitable for a detox. REMEMBER: For your ACV detox, choose foods as close to their natural state as possible, with no processed or dairy products.

It's important to approach any cleanse or detox regimen with caution and consult a healthcare professional before making significant changes to your diet or lifestyle. They can provide guidance based on your individual health needs and help you make informed decisions about your well-being.

ACV WEIGHT LOSS METHOD 3

Adding ACV Into Your Diet Plan to Lose Weight

Ok, here is the last of the 3 options for you to follow in order to lose weight using ACV.

Before we go onto this final method, let's just look quickly at some basic dietary advice as this will help you make the best decisions in your own meal planning attempts.

THE KEY TO LOSING WEIGHT AS FAST AS POSSIBLE IS TO MAKE SMALL CHANGES TO YOUR DIET.

If your weight is currently static (you're not gaining or losing weight) then you'll see the best results by cutting out between 200 – 300 kcals a day.

This is easily done by sacrificing any of your higher calorific treats such as a latte, cookies, bag of potato chips, candy bar etc.

If your diet doesn't contain any of these types of foods, then you'll need to look a little deeper and cut down on any excess fats or sugars you may be using.

If you're currently gaining weight, then you'll need to reduce your calories by more than this and adopt a new approach to eating by cutting out between 400 – 500 kcals a day.

Did you know that 1 in 3 people who diet, end up weighing more than when they first started? The main reason for this is because they choose crash diets which promise rapid weight loss, but ultimately lead to food deprivation. The dieter quickly becomes tired of the starvation diet and then binges on all of the forbidden foods. Any weight lost is quickly regained.

If you want long lasting results, you must stay well clear from any diet that...

- *Promises unrealistic weight loss*
- Is based on an off the wall or unbalanced eating program
- Tells you to eat certain amounts of some foods (like meat) in unlimited quantities but prohibits the consumption of others (like bread or fruits).
- These diets are unhealthy because they lack basic nutrients and can easily lead to eating disorders.

Here are the 6 key steps for a balanced diet:

Eat 5 smaller meals throughout the day	Don't skip meals - especially breakfast- and try not to leave your stomach empty for long periods, instead eat small, frequent meals that are easier to digest. Eat in moderation from all food groups (meats, fruits, veg, etc.)
Reduce your fat intake	Fat is the highest source of calories (9 calories per 1 gram). Avoid eating fried foods, instead boil or bake foods after removing any visible fat. Avoid cakes, pastries and pies, mayonnaise, cream, and dressings. Choose low-fat dairy products
Reduce the amount of sugar you eat	Sugar is added to many processed, pre-packaged foods. If you can't get by without it, try to have no more than 2 teaspoons of sugar a day and preferably use brown sugar
Eat plenty of fiber	Fiber helps to cleanse the digestive system and gives a feeling of fullness in the stomach which can reduce appetite. Eat whole meal bread instead of white
Eat less salt	Don't put extra salt in your food and don't keep it on the table when eating. Avoid foods with a very high salt content, like tinned or processed food or sauces
Keep a food diary	If you record everything you eat or drink for a week and then read it, you will realize a lot about your eating habits from doing this and maybe find where there are some hidden calories

It's very common to underestimate how much food we eat. Many people consume a lot more calories than they realise and end up feeling frustrated about not being able to lose weight. Often blaming their bad metabolism or family genes, but the truth is that what they really need to do is to reduce their portion sizes.

Remember this is a life-changing eating plan which will keep you healthy well into old age and the apple cider vinegar is going to boost your results from the moment you start. As well as seeing your waistline decrease, remember all those extras that come along with the ACV, making you look and feel better

The ACV Meal Plans

There are 2 options here. Firstly, you can use the following sample meal plans and adjust to include your own favorite healthy alternatives. You'll find loads of great recipes and meal ideas at the back of the book, split into breakfasts, lunches, dinners and snacks. There are at least 10 options in each section, so you have plenty to choose from

Or secondly you can use the second option which is the food exchange chart or use a combination of them both.

Let's start with the sample meal plans.

Sample ACV Meal Plans

There are so many different diets out there which all have their own benefits and drawbacks when it comes to weight loss. Talk to anyone who has ever tried losing weight and they'd be more than happy to tell you about the new fad diet they read about in some random blog or one recommended by their favourite fitness influencer.

This section will cover the basics of a traditional 3 meal a day weight loss meal plan, which incorporates ACV so that you have a better understanding of how to structure your food intake, depending on your dietary requirements. All meals and alternatives are merely a suggestion to provide you with an understanding of how to keep your diet varied and enjoyable.

Portion sizes should be adjusted for your needs, but remember, we often eat considerably more than we actually need. Try using smaller plates or bowls to trick your mind in to thinking you are eating the same amount, but actually serve yourself a little less.

On top of eating, you also need to be drinking 2 liters of water a day. Water is key for removing waste from the body, protecting your vital organs, maintaining a balanced environment (*homeostasis*), and keeping your joints lubricated - to name just a few.

You'll find all of the recipes in this section at the back of the book.

Vegetarian Sample Diet Plan

Morning Drink: Apple cider vinegar and water: Mix one to two tablespoons of ACV with a glass of water (8- 16 fl). You can adjust the ratio to suit your taste preferences. Some people also add a squeeze of lemon juice or a teaspoon of honey to enhance the flavor.

Meal #1 (Breakfast) Crunchy Nut Granola with Greek Yogurt

- *Vegan alternative: Coconut Yogurt*

Greek yogurt is a great source of probiotics. Probiotics are beneficial bacteria that support gut health and digestion. Greek yogurt undergoes a straining process that removes whey, resulting in a thicker consistency and higher protein content compared to regular yogurt. This process also helps concentrate the probiotics, making Greek yogurt an excellent choice for promoting a healthy digestive system and supporting overall gut health.

Meal #2 (Lunch) Indonesian Pineapple Salad with Dressing

- *Also suitable for Vegans*

Pineapple contains an enzyme called bromelain. Bromelain has been studied for its potential health benefits, including its anti-inflammatory properties. It is known to aid digestion, reduce post-workout muscle soreness, and support wound healing. This enzyme is found in highest concentrations in the core of the pineapple, so be sure to include it in your consumption for maximum bromelain intake.

Meal #3 (Dinner) Vegan Burritos with Black Beans

- *Also suitable for Vegans*

Black beans are a rich source of dietary fiber. A one-cup serving of cooked black beans provides approximately 15 grams of fiber, which is about 60% of the recommended daily intake. This high fiber content helps promote healthy digestion, aids in maintaining a healthy weight by promoting feelings of fullness and supports heart health by helping to lower cholesterol levels. Including black beans regularly in your diet can be a delicious and nutritious way to boost your fiber intake and support overall health.

Evening Drink: Fruit tea or green tea: Make a cup of green/fruit/herbal tea and let it cool slightly. Mix in one tablespoon of ACV and optionally add a squeeze of lemon or a teaspoon of honey/natural unsweetened maple syrup for added flavor.

Pescatarian Sample ACV Diet Plan

Morning Drink: Apple cider vinegar and water: Mix one to two tablespoons of ACV with a glass of water (8-16 fl oz). You can adjust the ratio to suit your taste preferences. Some people also add a squeeze of lemon juice or a teaspoon of honey to enhance the flavor.

Meal #1 (Breakfast) Spinach and Mushroom Frittata

Mushrooms are a natural source of vitamin D. While most vitamin D is obtained through sunlight exposure, mushrooms have the unique ability to produce vitamin D when exposed to ultraviolet (UV) light. This makes them one of the few non-animal food sources of this essential nutrient. By placing mushrooms in direct sunlight for a short period of time, their vitamin D content can significantly increase. Incorporating mushrooms into your diet can be a delicious way to boost your vitamin D intake, which is crucial for bone health, immune function, and overall well-being.

Meal #2 (Lunch) Spanish Prawns and a Mixed Leaf Salad

Prawns are a low-calorie and high-protein seafood option. Prawns are not only delicious but also provide numerous nutritional benefits. A 100-gram serving of prawns contains approximately 100 calories and packs around 25 grams of protein. This makes them an excellent choice for those seeking to meet their protein needs while keeping their calorie intake in check. Additionally, prawns are a good source of essential nutrients such as selenium, vitamin B12, and omega-3 fatty acids, which contribute to overall health and well-being.

Meal #3 (Dinner) Quick Thai Salmon Fishcakes

Salmon is a great choice for losing weight and maintaining overall health. The fatty nature of this fish makes it incredibly satiating and combining this with complex carbs provides you with a complete meal bursting with vitamins, minerals, and fibre.

Evening Drink: Fruit tea or green tea: Make a cup of green/fruit/herbal tea and let it cool slightly. Mix in one tablespoon of ACV and optionally add a squeeze of lemon or a teaspoon of honey/natural unsweetened maple syrup for added flavor.

Omnivore Diet ACV Sample Plan

Morning Drink: Apple cider vinegar and water: Mix one to two tablespoons of ACV with a glass of water (8-16 fl oz). You can adjust the ratio to suit your taste preferences. Some people also add a squeeze of lemon juice or a teaspoon of honey to enhance the flavor.

If meat is on your menu, following a balanced omnivore diet will provide you with the nutrients you need to lose weight and help your body to function optimally.

Meal #1 (Breakfast) Healthy Beans with Poached Eggs and Grilled Bacon

Whilst eggs provide a muscle-sustaining protein source, bacon can help replenish electrolytes due to its salty nature. Bacon also boasts one of the highest protein-to-fat balances whilst providing key vitamins and minerals such as magnesium, iron, niacin, riboflavin, and zinc. When eaten in moderation, bacon can be a highly satiating food due to its high fat and protein levels.

Meal #2 (Lunch) Apple Cider Vinegar Marinated Pork Chops

Pork is a rich source of thiamin (vitamin B1), which plays a vital role in converting food into energy and maintaining a healthy nervous system. Thiamin also supports cognitive function and helps regulate mood. Including pork in a balanced diet can contribute to meeting your thiamin requirements and support overall health and well-being.

Meal #3 (Dinner) Mediterranean Burgers

Consuming lean beef as part of a balanced diet can provide the body with a complete amino acid profile, aiding in the maintenance and development of lean muscle mass. Additionally, protein-rich foods like beef can help promote satiety, keeping you feeling fuller for longer and potentially supporting weight management goals.

Evening Drink: Fruit tea or green tea: Make a cup of green/fruit/herbal tea and let it cool slightly. Mix in one tablespoon of ACV and optionally add a squeeze of lemon or a teaspoon of honey/natural unsweetened maple syrup for added flavor.

Easy Option Diet

Alternatively, instead of being so rigid in your food selection, you can simply make choices based on selecting foods from each of the food types in the table below.

To have a healthy and balanced diet, you should ideally choose a food from each of the following lists to make each meal you have throughout the day.

- Eat a protein with a carbohydrate and a portion of vegetables.
- Each nutrient should be of equal size, about the amount you can hold in a cupped hand.

The lists don't include every possible option, but a good example is as follows…

CARBOHYDRATES	PROTEINS	VEGETABLES
Whole wheat pasta	Skinless chicken or turkey	Green leafy vegetables
Butternut squash	Fish – not battered or fried	Carrots
Brown rice	Shellfish	Broccoli
Baked or boiled potato	Egg whites	Tomatoes
Oats	Cottage cheese	Onions
Whole wheat bread	Low-fat yogurt	Mushrooms
Corn	Lean beef	Peppers
Barley or couscous	Semi or skimmed milk	Celery
Bulgar wheat	Tofu	Egg plant
Sweet potatoes	Quorn	Cauliflower
Quinoa	Beans and pulses	Peas

An example meal might be brown rice, chicken (baked in foil) and steamed broccoli. An example breakfast might be porridge made with milk and a homemade sugar-free fruit smoothie. Look at the recipes at the end of this book, which contain apple cider vinegar or alternatively drink the apple cider vinegar and water mix before each meal.

The key to changing your eating habits for the long term is to phase all these changes in slowly over a couple of months. Try to get the hang of maybe just drinking water in week 1. Then in week 2 you might decide to cut out pies, pastries, and puddings and so on.

REMEMBER THIS IS A LIFE-CHANGING EATING PLAN WHICH WILL KEEP YOU HEALTHY WELL IN TO OLD AGE

if you keep doing it.

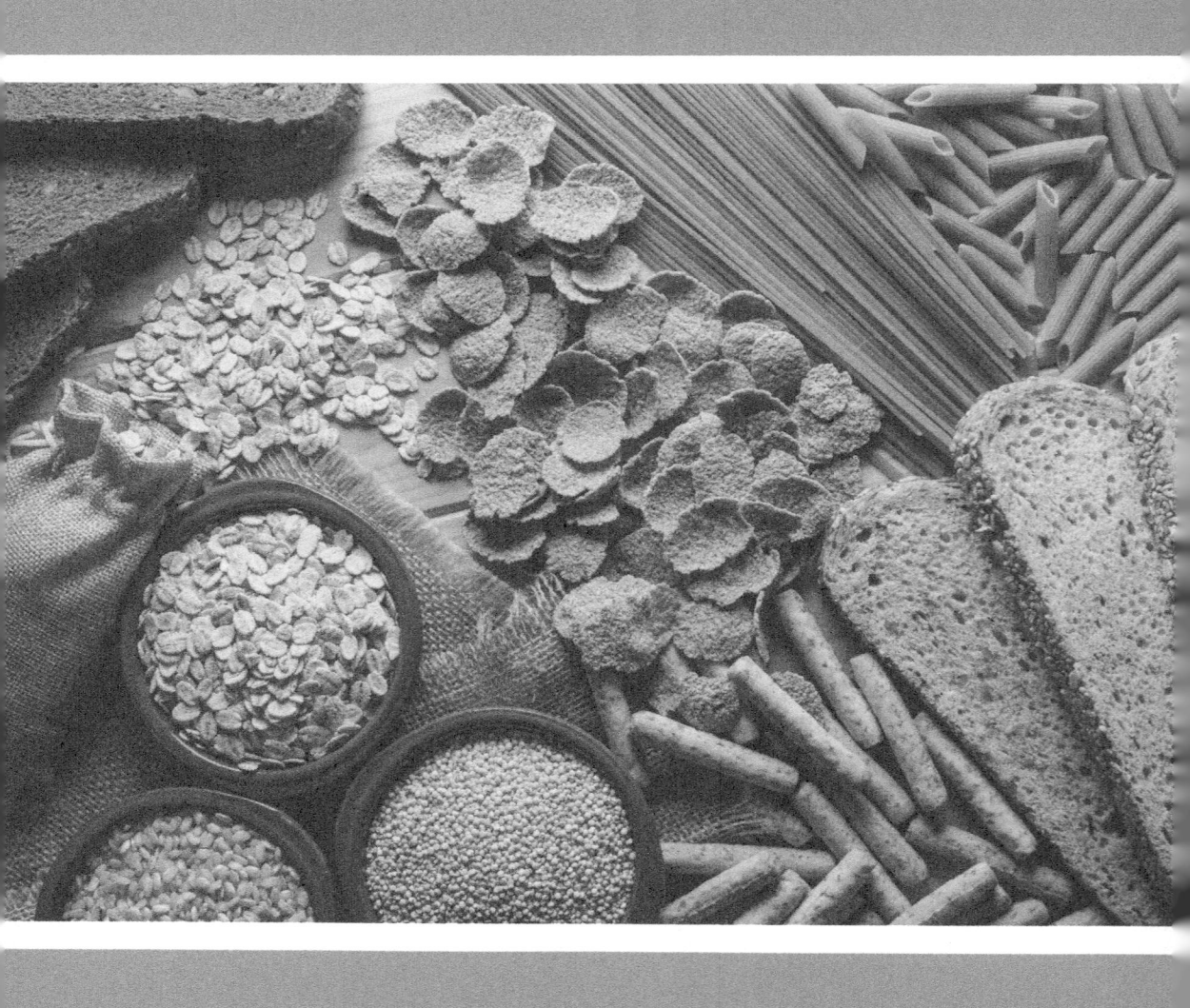

10 GOLDEN RULES OF WEIGHT LOSS

> Although apple cider vinegar is acidic, it has an interesting effect on the body. When consumed, it can actually help promote a more alkaline pH balance in the body. This is due to the way it is metabolized in the body, resulting in an alkaline effect. However, it is important to note that the impact on overall body pH may be minimal and can vary between individuals.

Here's a quick summary of the best ways of changing the way you eat and drink in order to lose weight...

Drink plenty of Water: Aim to drink at least 2 liters of fresh water a day.

Tip. Fill a 2-liter bottle and drink from that bottle all day. Doing this ensures that you know how much you have drunk. Water helps to cleanse the system and maintain hydration.

Eat more fruit and vegetables: You should aim to eat at least 5 portions of fresh fruit and vegetables each day. This total can include frozen fruit and vegetables or tinned ones in water or juice as opposed to sweetened syrup.

Tip. Always keep a fruit bowl handy and full of your favorite fruits.

Think natural: Try to eat foods that are as close to their natural state as possible with minimum processing.

Tip. Get into the habit of examining food labels, generally speaking the fewer ingredients added, the closer it will be to its natural state.

Always eat breakfast: After a night of sleep the metabolism slows right down – as you've not digested any food. Eating breakfast will kick-start the metabolism for the day and help you lose more weight.

Tip. Try a slice of toast with a thin spreading of no added sugar fruit spread immediately after waking.

Many people complain of a sickly feeling after eating in the morning, but this will disappear when the body is trained into accepting breakfast.

No food is a sin: By cutting out certain foods from your diet your body will crave them all the more. Choose one treat food and one or two days a week to have it and stick to this. Many highly processed foods are high in calories but low in nutritious bulk therefore you don't feel full after eating them and as a result eat more total calories.

Eat more wholegrain products: Eating wholegrain foods will give your diet the maximum natural goodness as possible, you will feel fuller after eating and your food will be digested more easily.

Tip. As a tasty nutritious snack why not try toasted wholemeal muffins with a little low-fat spread or for main meals use brown rice as the base.

Try to find healthy alternatives: Look at your favourite meals and try to find better ways of preparing them. Search for healthier take away options and less fatty restaurant foods.

Tip. Potato fries can be replaced by oven-baked potato wedges cooked in olive oil.

Experiment with foods: Try different foods - you might enjoy them. Eating a variety of foods will ensure you get a variety of vitamins and nutrients, which will make you feel healthier.

Tip. During your weekly shop aim to buy one new nutritious item and try one new recipe or meal each week.

Cut down on saturated fats: By reducing your intake of saturated fats you are doing one of the single most beneficial things you can do to improve your health.

Tip. Aim to become more aware of the fat content of foods and try to buy foods with minimal amounts or no saturated fats in the ingredient listings.

Don't listen to people who put you down: Decide on your goals and write them down. Don't listen to people who put you down or get in the way of you achieving your goals.

Tip. Find a picture of the way you would like to look and keep this on display - be realistic but be determined.

Don't forget the Apple Cider Vinegar: When the weight loss starts and you are feeling good, don't be tempted to forget the ACV, it could be making a bigger contribution to your weight loss and how much better you are feeling than you think! It might seem obvious, but don't stop doing something that works!

We have the power to change and shape our bodies in incredible ways.

REMEMBER FAILURE IS NOT FALLING DOWN ITS STAYING DOWN

So, when you slip up, get right back again, and renew your dedication to your goals.

MEASURING WEIGHT LOSS

If your aim is to lose weight or tone up, then you need to measure what is happening to your body and your overall shape to know if you're making progress.

It's very difficult to see changes in the mirror alone, and *most of us have a distorted image of how we actually look anyway*.

Weighing scales can tell you how much you weigh overall but probably won't accurately measure your progress. Because your weight is made up of bone, muscle, fat, and water. It's not good to lose water, it's definitely not good to lose muscle but it is good to lose body fat if you are storing too much of it.

When dieting or changing eating habits, a lot of the initial weight loss is often due to a loss in the amount of water in your body.

> **LOSING BODY FAT IS THE GOAL OF ANY WEIGHT LOSS PROGRAM AND ITS SUCCESS CAN ONLY BE MEASURED BY THE AMOUNT OF FAT LOST, NOT OVERALL WEIGHT.**

Once you start eating normally, water and weight will be gained back immediately as your body doesn't like being dehydrated; it affects the body's internal water balance and can actually slow down the metabolism.

Losing muscle is not good either because this also slows down the metabolic rate.

By taking measurements at regular intervals, you are doing two things. Firstly, you can see whether your current efforts are having an effect, if they are, keep doing what you are doing, if not make some changes. For example, you might be able to increase the amount of activity you are doing. Secondly it maintains your awareness and helps to keep you focused on your goals and objectives.

When measuring around the waist, don't tense or pull in your tummy muscles, just stand relaxed.

When measuring your hips, stand with your feet together. I suggest taking the measurement around the widest part and do this two or three times just to make sure that you've got it right.

Make sure that you can retake the measurement again in the same place the next time, so put the same amount of tension on the measuring tape.

Here are the most effective methods of monitoring your progress:

Take a photo	Take photos of yourself before you start. It's much easier to be objective when you look at a paper copy of yourself. Some people may find this a painful step, but it's an important process to help you stay motivated. Ideally you should take pictures wearing just your underwear, remember these are for your reference only. Taking shots from the front, back and both sides is the best way. Keep these photos near you and look at them regularly. This will keep you focused and drive you forward, particularly when you start to see changes.
Use a piece of clothing	A pair of trousers, a skirt, some shorts, or a dress can be a good guide to your progress. Try them on every now and then to see if you're making progress. If they feel tight to begin with that's ideal.
Use a tape measure	A simple tape measure found in sewing kits is probably one of the quickest and most practical ways of charting your progress. You should measure both around the hips and the waist to get a true indication of your progress.
How you feel	Ask yourself regularly each week how you feel. Score this from one to ten, ten being fantastic and one being awful. Make a record of this figure in your diary.
Get a body fat reading	If you have a gym membership, ask the staff there to take a body fat reading. The best and most reliable method of testing body fat levels and the loss of fat is by using skin fold calipers. All good gyms should be able to carry out this test for you quickly and reliably.

Another sign of healthy weight loss and an active lifestyle are your skin, hair, and nails. These virtually always look and feel better when you start to lose weight or become more active.

If you are still intent on judging your success by standing on a set of scales each week, bear in mind that you're only getting part of the picture.

> **The best way to monitor your progress is to use a combination of methods and never just rely on weighing scales alone**

APPLE CIDER VINEGAR SUPPLEMENTS

Commonly used in salad dressings, marinades, and pickling recipes. Its tangy flavor and acidic properties make it a versatile ingredient in the kitchen, adding a distinctive taste to dishes.

While it helps to include ACV in your diet by incorporating recipes that make use of this incredibly versatile ingredient, it is often recommended to take ACV on its own or with water, so you get the benefits of pure ACV right away.

Alternatively, you can buy apple cider vinegar capsules which are good if you're very sensitive to the taste of ACV but do try to take it in its natural form - even if you find it difficult to take. It will become easier over time. Many people enjoy the taste and feel of the ACV and are happy to take it, but everyone is different. Whatever your preferences, ACV will still benefit you in many ways.

Apple cider vinegar supplements are capsules or pills that contain concentrated amounts of apple cider vinegar (ACV) in powdered form. These supplements are designed to provide the potential health benefits of ACV in a convenient and easy-to-consume format. They are typically sold as dietary supplements in health food stores, pharmacies, or online.

Apple cider vinegar supplements aim to provide the same components found in liquid ACV, including acetic acid and other organic acids. These supplements may be marketed as a way to support weight loss, digestion, blood sugar control, or overall health. However, it's important to note that the scientific evidence supporting the effectiveness of apple cider vinegar supplements is limited and often preliminary.

It's crucial to choose ACV supplements from reputable brands and to follow the instructions provided on the product packaging. Dosage recommendations may vary among different brands, so always read, and adhere to the specific guidelines.

As with any dietary supplement, it's advisable to consult with a healthcare professional before you start taking it - especially if you have any underlying health conditions or are taking medications. They can provide personalized advice based on your individual health needs and help you determine whether apple cider vinegar supplements are suitable for you.

It's important to note that while apple cider vinegar supplements offer convenience, they may not provide the same benefits as consuming ACV in its liquid form.

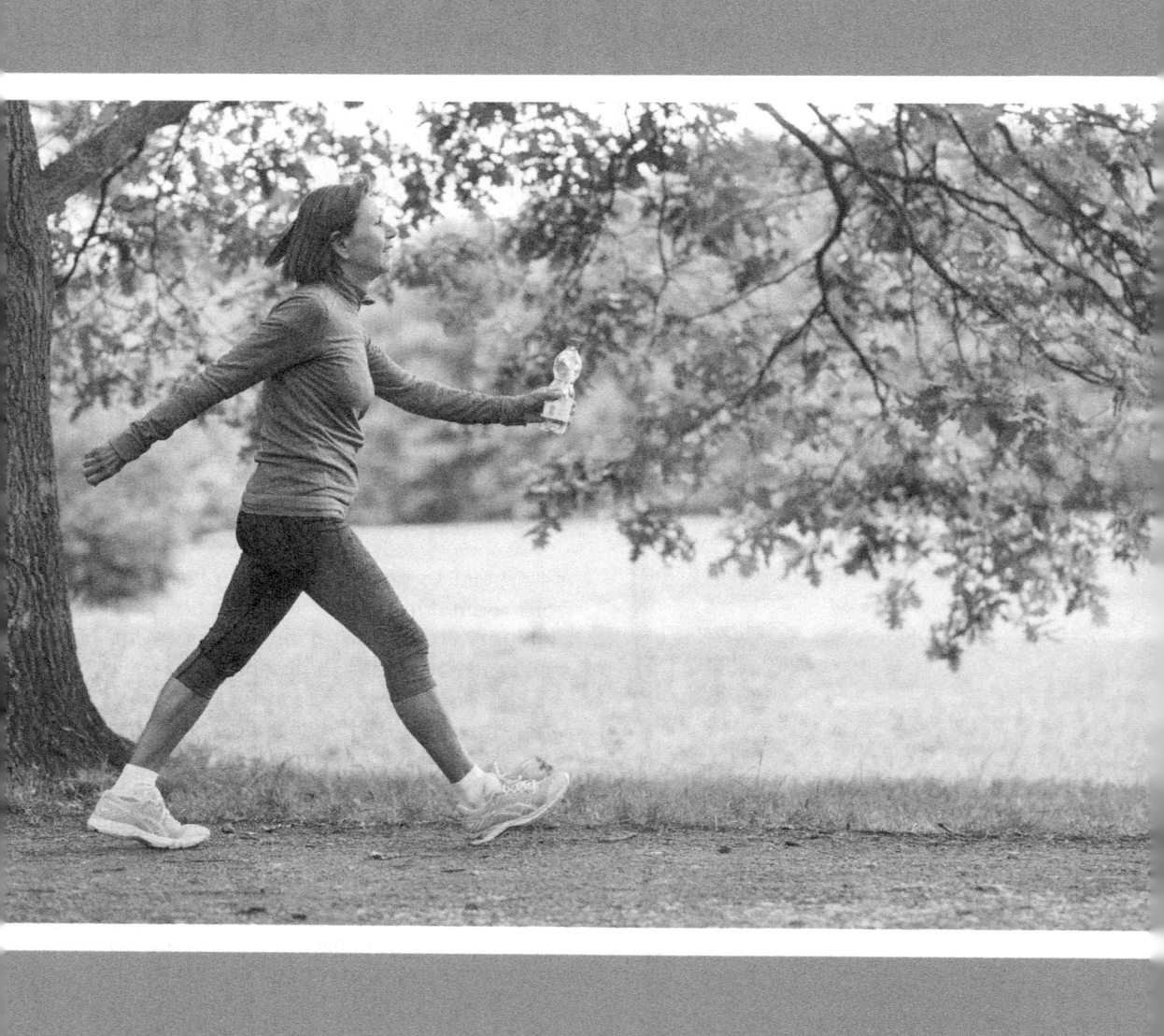

WHAT ABOUT EXERCISE?

> Apple cider vinegar is low in calories and contains trace amounts of beneficial compounds including acetic acid, which gives vinegar its characteristic tangy taste, and small amounts of amino acids, antioxidants, and polyphenols.

I was waiting for you to ask about that!

With any weight loss plan, it's essential to make the most of every tool in your toolbox and trying to lose weight without becoming more active is like trying to drive your car with one hand tied behind your back – much harder!

So, the key is to find something you can do easily and that fits in to your daily schedule, is free and works. Well, I have the answer for you here...

Walking

Two of the easiest and most effective changes you can make when embarking on a weight loss program (no matter how unfit or overweight you may consider yourself to be) are increasing your water intake and starting a walking program.

The vitality and wellness you get from taking ACV is going to stand you in perfect stead when it comes to boosting your activity levels. In the same way, increasing your walking by embarking on a regular walking program, and trying to fit in more movement and activity into your day is going to boost how effective the apple cider vinegar is.

Before we get into the details of setting your walking program, let's look at the benefits of walking.

Exercise through walking will give an incredible boost to your overall health; including improved heart health and weight loss, as well as beneficial changes in your mental wellbeing – how you feel on a day-to-day basis.

Walking regularly can improve your sleep (insomnia affects 55% of us). It can also help improve your overall energy levels. We all get times when we lack energy. Our lives are so busy – imagine if you could give yours a boost – without the sugary snacks.

You may believe that because walking isn't as high intensity as some other forms of exercise, that there aren't that many benefits compared to something like aerobics, however this is absolutely not the case.

Regular walking will help you to lose weight and can prevent disease and serious illness such as diabetes and arthritis. Walking regularly will improve your health, as well as reduce your risk of ill health. It will increase your overall muscle tone and bone density as well as lowering body fat levels. If you commit to a regular walking schedule, then you'll start to feel healthier and far less stressed.

Bearing in mind everything that you've just read, why wouldn't you want to walk?

If a miracle drug came along and promised all these benefits, you'd be taking it every day – so let's get walking!

Walking is an 'easy to do' activity that gives you the chance to work at a comfortable level of intensity, without the need to use expensive equipment or having to train in specific places. All these things make it the ideal choice for those wanting to become more active and lose weight.

Becoming fit and active is not just about going to a gym, fitness class or playing sport, it's more about beginning a new way of life so that exercise and activity becomes part of everyday life… something you just do without thinking about or planning it.

You need to change your outlook on life. Keeping joints supple, retaining muscle tone, maintaining a healthy heart and lungs and normalizing body weight and levels of body fat are all reasons why you should spend the time and effort it takes to walk regularly.

Walking can be an essential part of this process of change for these reasons: -

- Every able-bodied person can do some form of walking
- Walking is free, it doesn't cost anything
- Social groups can be based around the activity
- It can be done straight away after leaving the house, anywhere and at any time
- It can be done as part of a daily routine
- Puts very little stress on the bones and joints making it suitable for anyone that is overweight
- Improves the strength of the heart and lungs
- Can help you lose weight
- Can improve your fitness levels, giving you more energy and helping you to sleep better

To get the most out of walking you should design a route around where you live which will take you between half an hour and one hour to complete, in surroundings you feel comfortable with.

This route should be walked at a comfortable pace for the first few times and then done progressively faster so that you feel warmer, you are breathing slightly heavier and your heart rate increases. You should still be capable of holding a conversation.

Your route should include some gentle gradients if possible because these push the body to a greater degree than simply walking on the flat.

You should make a note of how difficult it feels on the first few attempts at your route as these feelings will quickly disappear when your fitness levels improve.

If fitness is your aim, you will need to regularly increase the speed at which you walk over a period of time.

If weight loss is your goal, then the more often you can get out and walk then the more calories you will burn. It is true that the more effort you put in, the faster results you'll get. But be patient and aim to progress slowly but steadily.

If you burn an excess of 3,500 kcals over your normal exercise and dietary requirements each week, then this will lead to a weight loss of approximately 1lb. Walking provides an excellent way of burning off those extra calories without having to do too much hard work.

Be careful when walking alone, be sure to let others know where you are walking to or use a route which is quite busy.

The footwear you choose should be comfortable and designed so that the heels are elevated slightly, also it's best to wear layers of thin clothing so that as the body temperature increases, these layers can be removed.

Try to avoid wearing thick heavy coats or oversized jumpers.

I recommend that you try to walk more every day. Aim to do at least 30 minutes although don't worry if you can't do all of this in one go. Breaking your walks down in to smaller chunks is still a very effective way of doing things.

Research confirms that shorter bouts of exercise, like walking, are just as effective when it comes to losing weight as longer periods. So, this means you could do 4 smaller 15-minute walks in a day and get the same results as walking for 60 minutes in one go.

And what's more, studies have shown that over the course of an hour of brisk walking it's possible to burn off more calories and lose more weight compared to jogging. The reason for this is that walkers take more steps and swing their arms more often than joggers.

If you make some small changes to the things you eat and walk regularly then walking really can have a dramatic effect on your weight loss.

Not only that but the health benefits of walking are dramatic too...

- Studies prove that walking one mile in 16 minutes lowers your cholesterol levels the same amount as running a mile in 7 - 10 minutes.

- **Walking is easier on your joints.** A walker's foot lands with only 1.5 times the force of body weight, whilst running on average puts three times the downward force on your feet.

- Walking just three hours a week cuts the risk of heart attack and stroke in women aged 40- 65 by 40% (Harvard Medical School).

- Women who walk 40 - 45 minutes five times a week are sick with colds or the flu half as often as sedentary women (Appalachian State University).

- Your weight loss from walking can be 18 pounds a year, without dieting, if you walk 45 minutes, four times a week (University of Massachusetts Medical School).

One of the key facts you should be aware of when considering whether to start a walking program or to try running instead is this...

Whilst you may well burn off more calories if you run for 30 minutes compared to walking for 30 minutes (if you can keep running for that long) but the fuel you use for both will be totally different.

When you run as a beginner and your heart rate increases to cope with the challenge, you're burning mostly sugar, or carbohydrates, which is how your body gives you fast energy in bursts. When you walk however, your body has the time to switch from burning carbohydrates to burning fat.

Remember walking does work, it's an extremely effective way of losing weight and toning up the whole of the lower body, but you must be consistent.

The following list of tips and strategies should help you to easily fit walking into your daily routine. Even on your busiest days you'll find suggestions that you can use to get at least some walking done.

Here are my suggestions which I have grouped in to 5 different categories…

General Walking Tips

1. Be Safe. Walk in familiar, well-lit areas. Carry a mobile phone with you just in case you need any help.

2. Use your mobile phone and listen to your favorite tracks or motivational or inspirational podcasts as you go

3. If you wear headphones, earbuds, or pods, make sure you keep the volume level low enough so you can still hear what's happening around you.

4. Get your arms involved. You'll burn more calories and walk much faster if you swing your arms when you walk.

5. When out shopping, why not do a couple of laps of the mall or shopping center first, to make up for the coffee you'll have later!

6. Keep a track of everything you do. Recording your activities and the foods you eat can help to motivate you to keep going and making progress.

7. Try a few different walking routes so you don't get bored. Keep a record of the times it takes you to do each one and then once a week pick one of your routes and aim to beat your best time.

8. How about trading calories for steps so let's say you've been out for a meal, and you had a dessert, why not work out how many calories it contained and then walk it off the next day?

9. Try to maintain your new walking regime for at least a month so that it becomes more of a habit without the need for you to think about it.

10. Walk faster. Whenever you can, try to take quicker steps, instead of longer ones. Longer and quicker steps will make you faster, quicker steps will help you to burn more calories.

11. Remember how much good you're doing for your health by walking, and enjoy the scenery, stores, and people you see whilst you're doing it.

12. If you've missed a few walks because you've been away, too busy, or not very well, don't worry about it, just start again whenever you can. The sooner you get back into the exercise groove the better.

13. When going on holiday, choose one where you'll have plenty of opportunities to walk, for instance along a beach or in the countryside etc.

14. Don't take the car for short journeys, walk there instead, you'll get in more exercise, burn more calories, AND save money.

15. When shopping why not park as far away as possible from the store as this is a really good way to get in more steps. Also, the funny thing is everyone else wants to park as close as possible, so there should be many more parking spaces available for you to choose from.

16. Treat yourself to some walking gear. Spending your money on this may motivate you to use it and walk more often.

17. Contact local walking associations and join in their organized walking sessions.

18. Walk at different times of the day, the things you'll see first thing in the morning for example, will be very varied and completely different to the ones you'll see at other times.

19. Make walking part of the occasion, so if you're going out for a meal, why not choose somewhere within walking distance and walk there and back. Doing this means, you'll certainly lessen the effects of the dessert if you had one.

20. If it's not pouring down with rain, why not walk the first or last part of your journey or if you go by bus, get off a few stops early.

21. Go for a walk during your lunch break, walk to get your lunch or to find somewhere to eat your lunch.

Walking At Home

1. Walk to the nearest store instead of driving or popping in on your way home

2. Most of your walking can be part of your everyday routine, for example, walking around when you're on the phone, getting off the bus early or walking to school or college.

3. Walk the dog, if you don't have one yourself, borrow a neighbor's dog or get in touch with a rescue center to help them out too. If you're expected to be there every day, you're far more likely to turn up and do your walks.

4. Treat yourself to a treadmill. Ok, you might not have the space or the money to buy one, so if not, you could always go to the gym or borrow a friends. This way you won't have any excuses if the weather gets bad or it's very late at night.

5. Get up and move around, do something active instead of lounging on the couch for hours at a time in the evenings.

6. Get up early in the morning to do your walk at this time. Everywhere looks so much different in the early hours, you feel like the world is yours and you'll set yourself up for a great day.

7. Why not cancel your morning deliveries such as the newspapers or milk and go and collect them yourself.

8. If you ever run short of supplies, walk to the store to buy them instead of taking the car.

9. Why not challenge yourself to walk up and down the stairs a certain number of times throughout the day.

10. If you have two bathrooms in the house, always use the upstairs one during the daytime.

11. Instead of channel hopping during commercial breaks, why not get up and walk around? You'll save getting bored, being programed to buy something you don't really need anyway, and you'll also get a little fitter in to the bargain.

12. If you're using a phone app or fitness watch to measure your walks, you can make up any shortfall of steps at home in the evening by walking around the house... walking is walking after all!

13. Did you realize that doing something as simple as changing the channels on the TV could really make a difference to your health? In fact, if you did this over a year, you'd actually lose weight too.

Walking At Work

1. Get yourself a tracking app or fitness watch and record how many steps you take each day. You can then set yourself mini targets to reach and have competitions with your family, friends, or colleagues at work.

2. Walk to the local grocery store to buy your lunch

3. Walk to work or park your car in the space that is the furthest away and walk to the office

4. During your work breaks get up and go for a walk around the block. You'll get more exercise and clear your head... you'll be far sharper and get more done when you get back to work.

5. If you need to speak to somebody in the office, walk over to them instead of phoning them.

6. Instead of sending emails to colleagues at work, get up and go over to talk to them, you'll be burning more calories and socializing at the same time.

7. Don't take the elevator - use the stairs instead.

8. A great way to unwind after a day at the office is by going out for a walk. Furthermore, walking with someone else and chatting can really help to solve the day's problems the stresses of everyday life.

9. Get off the bus early and walk the rest of the way home or to work.

10. Walk to the station instead of taking the car or bus.

Walking With Friends

1. Plan to go for a power walk once or twice a week with a friend.

2. If you arrange to meet friends, walk to their house, or get them to walk and meet you halfway.

3. Offer to join a friend or neighbor when they walk their dog.

4. Rather than meeting your friends for coffee, suggest going out for a stroll instead.

5. Find a walking partner so you have someone to chat to as you walk.

6. Make it a social thing, walk with a group of friends, or join or set up your own walking group.

7. Plan a route so that you can visit friends or family along the way.

Walking With Children

1. Walking is good for growing bones and muscles so walking regularly helps your children to grow up to be fit and strong.

2. Walk the children to the nearest playground or play center instead of driving there.

3. Find the time for one walk each week with each of your children - make this your special time when the two of you are alone and you can chat and catch up with things going on in their lives.

4. Plan fun exploration walks for the kids - get out and explore your local neighborhood.

5. Make it your mission to plan a new walk for each weekend - look out for local parks, country walks or nature trails etc.

6. If you drop your children at clubs / parties, don't spend the time driving back and forth, go for a walk yourself instead.

7. Get the whole family involved, make it fun for the kids. A picnic is a great idea to treat them when you reach your destination.

8. Set up a treasure hunt, so they must search for clues to track down the treasure... don't forget to leave them a treat at the end of it though!

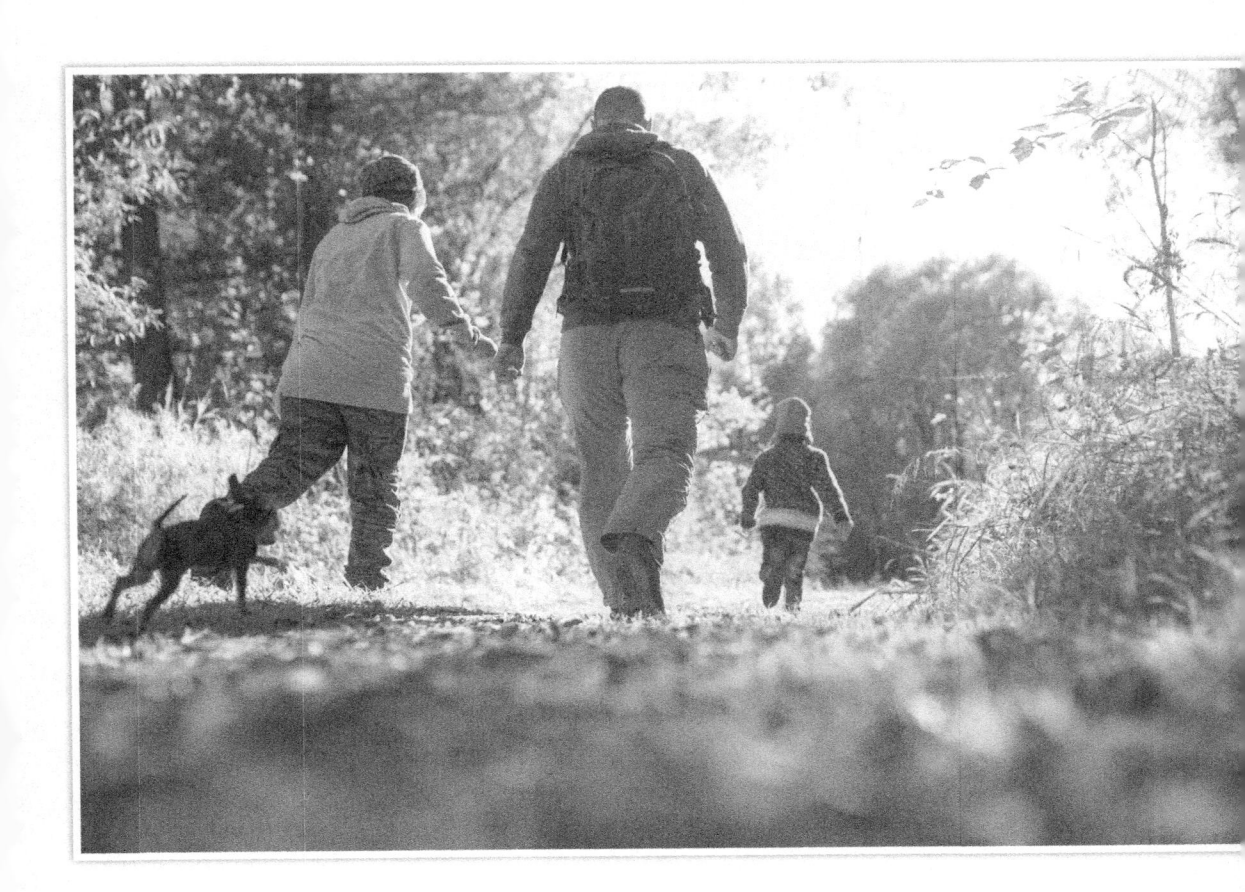

9. Why not go on a nature trail, get them to collect different colored wildflowers or work through the alphabet by finding a plant, insect, leaf, or flower beginning with the letter 'A' then 'B', 'C' etc.

10. Walk to the park. Take a frisbee or ball out with you and you'll get the chance to burn more calories still, plus the kids can get rid of some of that excess energy.

11. Walk the children to school - whatever the weather.

12. Stop off halfway at the park if you are walking with kids/dogs so they can have a play and a run around.

Using an App or Fitness Watch to Track Your Walking Steps Each Day

On average a typical person will walk approximately 3,000 – 4,000 steps each day, less if they have a particularly inactive job.

1,000 steps are the equivalent of walking for approximately 10 minutes.

A pedometer, fitness watch or phone app that tracks the number of steps you take each day is a step counting tool that will measure every step you take around the house, across the office, window shopping at the mall or going to school or the park.

Phone apps track the number of steps you take using the built-in sensors within your smartphone, typically an accelerometer or a combination of sensors including an accelerometer, gyroscope, and magnetometer.

Some apps allow users to calibrate or personalize step tracking based on their stride length or other individual characteristics. This involves inputting information such as height, weight, and gender to improve the accuracy of step counts. Calibration can help fine-tune the algorithm's calculations to better match your own individual stride length and walking pattern.

It's worth noting that while phone apps can provide a convenient way to estimate step counts and overall activity levels, they may not be as accurate as dedicated fitness trackers or pedometers. Factors such as phone placement, sensitivity of the sensors, and app algorithms can influence the accuracy of step tracking.

For sustainable weight loss, you should aim for a calorie deficit - that is, more calories used than consumed - of around 500 calories per day. Walking 10,000 steps more or less gets you to this total.

Taken over a week, this would mean you would have burned off a total of 3,500 kcals which is the amount needed to burn off 1lb of fat.

1lb per week is a very sustainable rate of weight loss because it is easily doable and unlikely to result in a weight gain rebound if you stop walking for any reason.

Using a pedometer or app to measure the number of steps you take in a day is a good way to start a physical activity program and a great way to track your progress.

Walking can also transform your health. Experts now say that taking roughly 10,000 steps per day sets off a chain reaction of physical benefits, including lowering blood pressure, reducing risk for heart disease, and bettering the odds for preventing breast cancer.

If 10,000 sounds like a lot, then you should break it down into smaller chunks of say 15-minute stints. Or why not get up from your desk or couch every hour and walk for 5 minutes instead.

10,000 steps converts to walking approximately 4.5 to 5 miles.

Keep up your new regime for a year and you could end up losing a whopping 52lbs – without the need to diet.

Basic Walking Weight Loss Plan

WHO'S IT FOR?

This program is ideally suited to the following people: -

- Anyone that is new to fitness and is currently inactive
- Anyone who is overweight
- Anyone who is trying to lose weight.
- Anyone who is recovering from injury.
- Any elderly or very young exercisers.

Workout Goals

To successfully complete a 3 mile/ 5-kilometer circuit by walking all the way without stopping.

Workout Duration

The program is based over 6 weeks.

Specific Workout Notes and Guidelines

When embarking on any new form of exercise which involves the repetitive movement of certain joints over extended periods of time - such as walking - it is vital that you ensure that the footwear you select is appropriate for your needs.

Running shoes are perfect for road or track walking etc. but if you intend to do any of your training off road using tracks, paths, over grass, sand, or mud, it will be a good investment to spend some extra money on a good pair of walking boots. The reason for this is that they have a much higher support around the ankle which helps to protect and stabilise the joint against any slight deviations in foot fall and walking surfaces.

The risks of you suffering from injuries due to your walking are far less likely than if you were training to run the distance, so you won't need to take as much rest in between workouts. But if you are quite overweight then the risk to your knees, lower back and ankles is still quite considerable, so you will need to listen to your body and be aware of any aches, pains and niggles you may feel.

During your sessions an ache in the muscles is to be expected - especially if you're walking up a gradient or using bursts of speed throughout your walks, in fact we actually want this type of reaction from the body.

What we don't want is any sharp or shooting pains, if you feel any of these, you should stop immediately to investigate the problem further.

Unless specified, select routes for your sessions that contain no hills or just slight gradients for your first few walks or any of the gentle walks listed in the program.

Gentle Walk

A gentle walk is meant to be performed at a comfortable pace, do not push yourself too hard during these sessions. In the program where the gentle walk is written as '2 x 10 minutes' for example, this means that you should perform two short walks at different times of the day, not immediately after each other.

Power Walk

This is brisk walking at a fast pace, trying to maintain a constant speed. You should start to sweat slightly, and your breathing will be constantly raised. The level of effort should be quite challenging.

Cross Training

This section of the program is meant to provide aerobic training to improve the strength and endurance of the heart and lungs at the same time as resting the muscles and joints used during walking. I recommend swimming, cycling, fitness DVD's or circuit training etc. Basically, anything which doesn't use the same mechanics as walking.

Hill Walk

Select any hills or inclines nearby to perform this session on. The aim during these workouts is to build up strength in the leg muscles and the heart and lungs. You should spend the allotted time actually walking up the hill, so the total time for a session wouldn't include the amount of time you spent walking downhill for example. If you don't have access to any hills, try using an inclinable treadmill or if you aren't able to use one, you can power walk instead.

Interval Training

There are two interval sessions in this program and for these you will use three different levels of intensity and speed as follows:

Gentle walking, brisk walking, and power walking. You can either choose to use landmarks for your intervals such as lamp posts or markers in the road for example, or alternatively use a stopwatch to time one-minute intervals at each speed.

Sunday Sessions

Once a week you will need to develop your endurance by performing some longer walks so that you build up to 5 kilometers without rest. You can of course choose any day to do this, but to suit the program and fit in rest days, I have structured Sundays as this day.

Basic Walking Plan

WEEKS	MONDAY	TUESDAY	WEDNESDAY	THURSDAY	FRIDAY	SATURDAY	SUNDAY
1	Gentle walk 10 minutes	REST	Gentle Walk 2 x 10 minutes	REST	Gentle Walk 20 minutes	REST	Gentle Walk 1 mile/1.6km
2	Cross Training 15 minutes	REST	Gentle Walk 2 x 15 minutes	REST	Hill Walk 10 minutes	REST	Walk 1½ miles/2.4km
3	Cross Training 20 minutes	REST	Gentle Walk 2 x 20 minutes	REST	Interval Training 25 minutes	REST	Walk 2 miles/3.2km
4	Cross Training 30 minutes	REST	Walk 30 minutes	REST	Hill Walk 15 minutes	REST	Gentle Walk 2½ miles/4km
5	Cross Training 35 minutes	REST	Power Walk 35 minutes	REST	Interval Training 30 minutes	REST	Walk 3 miles/4.8km
6	Cross Training 45 minutes	REST	Walk 45 minutes	REST	Hill Walk 30 minutes	REST	Brisk Walk 3½ miles/5.6km

What About Exercise

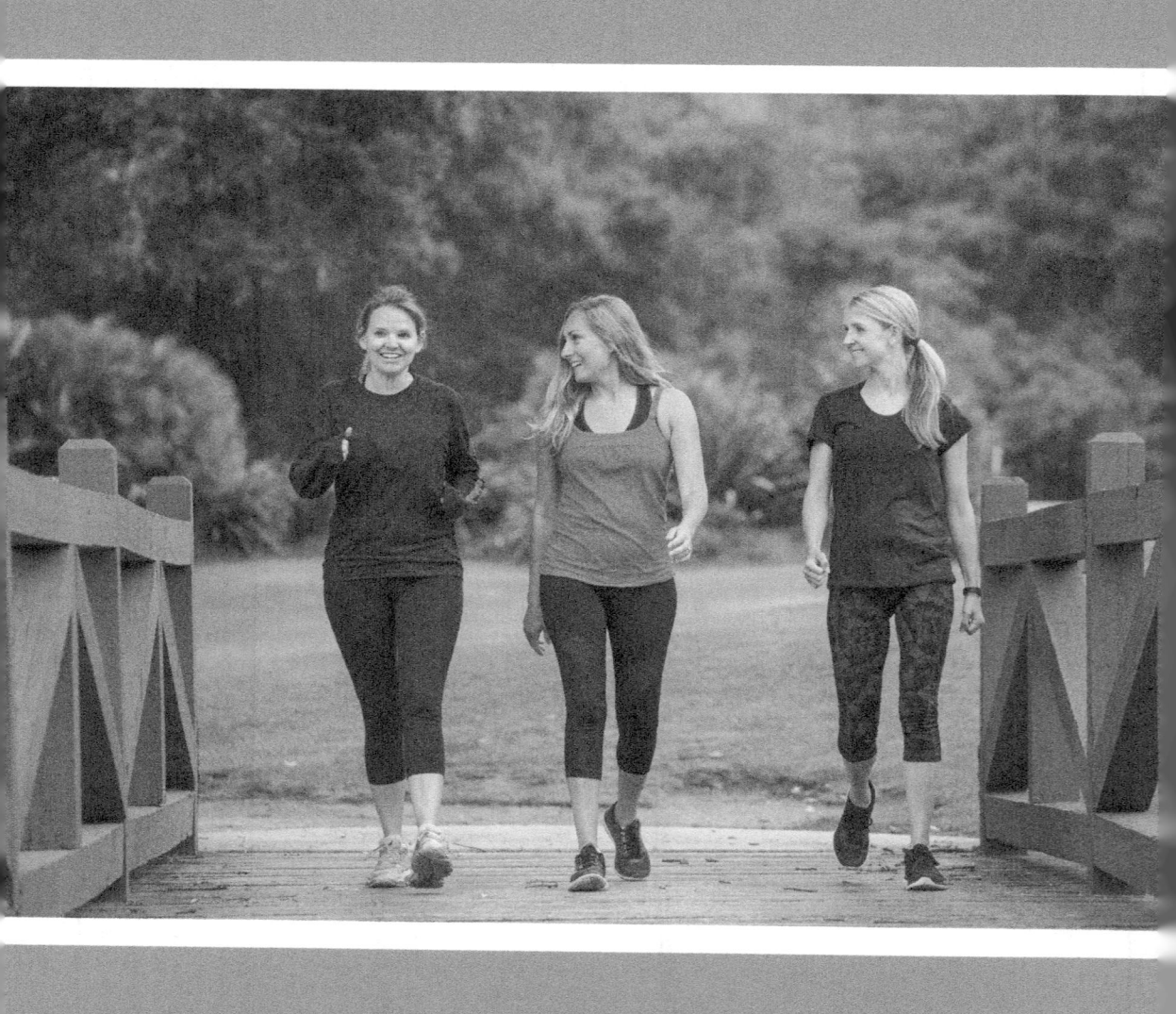

WALKING AND WEIGHT LOSS – THE FACTS

> Apple cider vinegar can be diluted with water and used as a facial toner to help balance the skin's pH level and reduce acne-causing bacteria. Additionally, it may be used as a natural hair rinse to enhance shine.

Clearly you want to lose weight and you're determined and ready to get started. You know you need to do some activity as well as improve your diet, so why not join a gym?

Most people think joining a gym is the quickest and easiest way to get fit, but this is far from true. You only need to look at gyms in early January and then again at the end of February to see that gyms don't work for most people.

The problem with joining a gym is that firstly you're going to need to pay a lot of money each month, and it's easier to join than to quit. Gym membership subscriptions are generally taken out of your bank account every month until your contract term expires. This is a fantastic business model for the gym because they know that once they've hooked customers in, they can then keep billing them until the customer ends the contract or at the end of the term.

Unless you use the gym regularly and enjoy the experience, you won't get your money's worth, and you may even feel like you've failed.

THE SECRET TO LOSING WEIGHT IS TO MAKE SURE THAT YOU TAKE PART IN ACTIVITIES THAT YOU ENJOY. So, if you find it boring at the gym, it's unlikely to work for you.

Why not try your local salsa dancing class, how about swimming, or even a local self-defence group instead? Pick something that gets you moving, motivated and suits your fitness levels. However, you can't say you don't enjoy something until you've tried it. So, keep an open mind and find a fun activity.

As we discussed in 'Goal Setting' another key to success is to have a plan of action, something written down that you can look at regularly. It's important that you commit to your goals and targets, instead of simply keeping them in your head. It's even better if you tell someone else about your plans - perhaps a close friend who can help keep you on track.

The brilliant thing about walking is that it suits all abilities, it's low impact (there's less risk of an injury), there's no special equipment needed, and IT WILL definitely **help you to lose weight if you commit to a regular plan**.

The key with walking is to be consistent. If you combine it with a healthy diet and ACV, you'll be amazed at the results. Every time you move around, you're walking and burning off calories. So, to lose weight you need to reduce your intake of calories a bit and increase the number of calories you burn off – it's as simple as that.

The more time you spend moving around then the more weight you'll lose.

How Many Calories Do You Burn Whilst Walking?

Any type of movement or activity burns off calories, and the more challenging the exercise, then the more calories you'll burn off. Exercises that involve moving the arms and legs at the same time will usually burn off more calories than doing either in isolation, which is another reason why walking is such a fantastic exercise because you can involve your arms at the same time as using the legs.

There are lots of ways to make walking more challenging (and therefore use up more calories) such as using hand weights, walking up hills or walking faster for short bursts of time.

In order to burn off 1lb of body fat, you need to use 3,500 calories more than you eat and drink.

This might seem like a huge number of calories, but if we take this over a week, then it's only **500 calories per day.** (Which is the equivalent to a fast-food burger or two slices of pizza)

> **REDUCING CALORIES IS BEST ACHIEVED THROUGH A COMBINATION OF BOTH DIET AND EXERCISE.**

So, if you take out your favorite high fat/sugar snack each day at around 200 – 300kcals (e.g., choosing an Americano coffee instead of a Latte) AND you become more active then you will begin to see very quick changes indeed.

There are a number of factors involved in burning off calories through walking, such as how long you walk for, how much you weigh, how fast you walk, and your current fitness levels etc.

The chart below can be used as a guide, this shows how many calories an average person weighing around 168lbs would burn over the space of one hour walking at different speeds.

These are only estimates, but the following chart should help you to understand the link between the effort you make - or time

Time	3mph (brisk walk)		4mph (fast walk)	
	Distance	Calories	Distance	Calories
10 minutes	0.5 miles	54 kcals	0.65 miles	64 kcals
30 minutes	1.5 miles	163 kcals	2 miles	193 kcals
60 minutes	3 miles	327 kcals	4 miles	386 kcals

spent walking - and the number of calories you will burn off.

If you add any hills or inclines to the speeds below, you can dramatically increase the number of calories - and therefore fat that you'll burn.

Committing To Changing Your Lifestyle

You've proven that you're committed to making a change in your life and you've clearly been thinking about this – otherwise you wouldn't be reading this guide.

However, I know from years of experience as a weight loss coach, that wanting to make a change and actually making that change are two totally different things.

So here are a few thoughts about starting off the right way and getting motivated...

Visualisation: The first thing I want you to do is to think about *what this change to your lifestyle will look and feel like* – fast forward 6 - 12 months ahead and imagine where you will be, what you'll be doing, how you'll look and how you'll feel as a result of your lifestyle change.

This might sound a little strange, but visualising where you want to be is essential. How can you plan your journey if you don't know where the end is... sports stars use this all the time to help them focus and to be successful.

You shouldn't go off into the realms of fantasy here, try not to think about magazine images... think of an improved you. Think of your friends commenting on *'how good you look these days'*, think about going to the shops and picking up clothes one size smaller... about feeling healthy and full of energy.

Preparing for a Change

Humans are programmed to take the easiest possible route in life, and we're also programmed to eat more than we need. So, to make a lifestyle change to get fitter and to lose weight may feel like you're working against your natural instincts at

> "Humans are programmed to try and find the easiest possible route in life, and we're also programmed to eat more than we need. So, to make a lifestyle change to get fitter and lose weight may feel like you're working against your natural instincts at first. You need to prepare for this and be tough with yourself."

first. You need to prepare for this and be tough with yourself.

One of the best pieces of advice I ever had when starting out on changing my lifestyle was to 'never switch off'. You always have to be thinking about what activities you need to do, and you always need to be thinking about what you're eating that day.

If you don't get tough with yourself, no one else will.

YOU NEED TO TAKE RESPONSIBILITY FOR THE ACTIONS AND CHOICES YOU MAKE IN LIFE.

Everyone has setbacks. When you've invested so much into a change of lifestyle, as you will have done, any setback can seem overwhelming. You may be surprised by how emotional you get. However, *don't let any setbacks defeat you*. This is the time to get a supportive friend round or on the 'phone and have a good natter about what's on your mind. **It's time to remember how much you achieved so far.**

The main thing is to follow the famous phrase 'Keep calm and carry on', don't let a setback throw out your whole program, if you have a bad day or even a bad week, remember the images of the future you and get back on track. If you get an injury or can't walk, then try swimming instead – do something else, even housework is quite good for fitness. Keep positive and you'll survive through the tough times.

Drinking Water for Weight Loss and Health

Aim to drink 2 liters of water every day. This might seem counter-intuitive if you are using apple cider vinegar to try to get rid of fluid you are retaining, but there are several reasons why you should drink this amount of water each day; having plenty of water ensures that several things happen which complement the actions of ACV in the body...

- Nutrients are assisted in their transportation around the body

- The digestive system is lubricated, and the correct body temperature is maintained

- Toxins are removed from the body. These are often stored just below the skin's surface in the form of cellulite and other fatty tissues.

- Fluids lost through everyday activities – and more especially during exercise- can be replaced immediately, thereby avoiding dehydration.

- Total level of body fat is reduced because water thins out the fatty acids which are used in the body for energy, or if they are not needed immediately, they are stored for future use.

- Dehydration is avoided which can cause the metabolism to slow down. The opposite is also true in that when there is adequate water in the body, the metabolism is speeded up.

Water is the most essential substance needed by the body... thirst should not be used as an indicator of the body's fluid status because at this point, you are probably already dehydrated.

Don't wait until you are thirsty before you drink.

Water, milk, and sugar-free drinks can all be counted as part of your daily water consumption. Fruit juices and sugary drinks are termed as *hypertonic* – this means they have a higher concentration of sugar than the blood and therefore cannot be absorbed into the bloodstream to assist in maintaining normal fluid levels. If you enjoy fruit juice as part of a balanced diet, try diluting it with water to better hydrate your body.

Try keeping a 2-liter bottle of water in the refrigerator and drink from this each day to ensure you are drinking the correct amount. Alternatively keep a few ½ liter bottles in the fridge, car, bedroom etc.... this ensures there is always water on hand, and they act as a gentle reminder.

As an alternative to plain tap or bottled water, try adding ice, lemon, or lime to give a refreshing alternative. Occasional use of carbonated water also gives an added twist. Check flavored water has no added sugar and drink occasionally as an alternative.

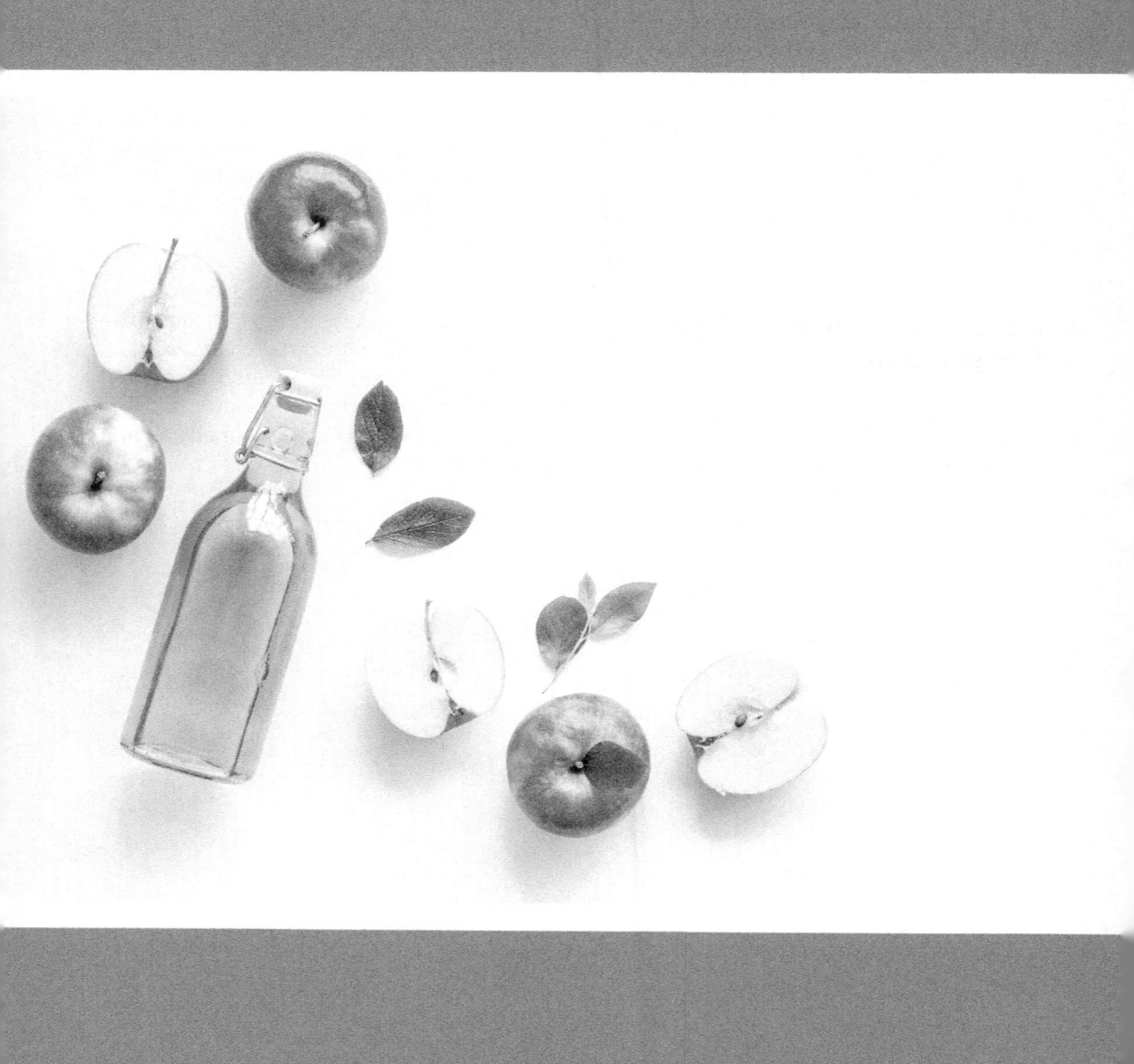

USING APPLE CIDER VINEGAR IN YOUR BEAUTY REGIME

> Apple cider vinegar can be diluted with water and used as a facial toner to help balance the skin's pH level and reduce acne-causing bacteria. Additionally, it may be used as a natural hair rinse to enhance shine.

Keeping a bottle of ACV in your bathroom may seem strange, but its wide range of uses in helping to keep you looking good as well as feeling good means it's a great choice for bathing, cleansing, and dealing with those irritating beauty concerns. It is considerably cheaper than expensive treatments, and when it goes down the plug, it isn't releasing dangerous chemicals into the water supply and into the environment; in fact, it is cleaning your plumbing!

Cleansing Detox Bath

This bath will draw out toxins, ease aches and pains and help with cramps and that feeling of tiredness you sometimes get in your feet and legs after a long hard day. Simply add one cup of apple cider vinegar, ½ cup of sea salt and one cup of Epsom salts to a tub of hot water and soak your cares away. Follow this up with a refreshing cool shower or body brush and feel renewed vigor!

Squeaky Clean Hair Rinse

Use a mixture that is half ACV and half water to create an invigorating scalp and hair rinse. It gets rid of dandruff, removes all traces of hair products and leaves hair squeaky clean. A quick rinse with water afterwards will eliminate any vinegar odor and your hair will be clean and shiny with a clear scalp.

To Deter Head Lice

Head lice and nits can be tough to get rid of, and some of the products on the market are very strong. If your child has head lice, or if you find them in your own hair, try dabbing the scalp with apple cider vinegar to deter the bugs. The same technique can help protect you from catching head lice if someone close to you has them.

> "One of the best pieces of advice I can give you when starting out on a weight loss diet is 'never switch off.' You always have to be thinking about what exercise or activity you can do that day, and what you're going to eat. If you leave these things to chance, you're setting yourself up to fail."

Cooling Astringent

To create your own natural cleanser for oily skin, use one cup of apple cider vinegar in 2 cups of cool water. Gently wipe a cotton ball dipped in the mixture over the skin. Rinse well. Use this morning and night for very oily skin, or every few days for combination skin.

Say Goodbye to Ugly Calluses

A callus is an area of thick skin that builds up over time due to pressure or rubbing, particularly over the hands. Apple cider vinegar can help soften and reduce calluses on hands and feet. Just add a cup of apple cider vinegar to a foot bath or hand bath and allow your skin to soak for 10 - 15 minutes before gently removing the calloused areas with a pumice stone and then applying hand or foot cream.

USING APPLE CIDER VINEGAR IN THE HOME

Unlike many other food products, apple cider vinegar has an incredibly long shelf life. Due to its high acidity, it has natural preservative properties, which means it can last indefinitely without spoiling.

Not only is ACV a potent and versatile thing to have in your bathroom cupboard and medicine cabinet, but it is also a fantastic product to add to your hoard of cleaning supplies. In fact, a few bottles of apple cider vinegar could go a long way to replacing a lot of what you normally use to keep your home clean and fresh.

Here are a few clever ways you can use ACV in and around your home…

Rid Your Home of Fleas

No-one likes to admit when fleas have taken hold of their home, but if you have pets, it is sometimes difficult to prevent the odd occurrence of fleas.

Apple cider vinegar can help rid your pet of fleas in an environmentally friendly manner, without any of the harsh chemicals that are found in commercial flea treatments.

Simply mix 2 parts ACV with one part water and rub thoroughly into the animal's coat.

General Household Cleaning

Mix 1 part apple cider vinegar with 2 parts warm water and use the mixture to clean surfaces such as worktops, tiles, floors, and kitchen surfaces. This is an especially good cleaning solution for areas where you don't want to use harsh chemicals, for example on children's toys and highchairs, or around animals.

Powerful De-Odorizing

Apple cider vinegar is great at neutralizing odors and ridding surfaces of lingering smells. This is ideal for surfaces or fabrics (always check for colorfastness) that have been moldy or that have had mildew. That dank, musty smell can linger even after the mold itself is gone.

Not only will a solution of 1 part ACV and 1 part water get rid of this unpleasant smell, but it will also kill off any remaining mold spores and make the problem less likely to re-occur - especially if you allow the vinegar to dry in the sunlight.

To prevent mold regrowth on walls or surfaces; simply wipe over the area with this same solution every so often to avoid the problems happening again.

Clear Those Drains

This is a great way to clear outdoor drains which are slow moving or blocked. To use this for an indoor basin, use a much smaller amount to avoid a mess! This is quite a fun solution to mix because it incorporates baking soda along with the vinegar which results in a bubbling reaction as carbon dioxide is released. First put ½ cup salt into the drain, then a cup of baking soda and follow this with a cup of ACV. Allow it to work its magic for two hours before flushing with plenty of water.

Remove Lime Scale

The acetic acid in the vinegar is ideal for removing lime scale build-up on water taps, use it neat to remove limescale and rinse well for a gleaming finish. Rinse with water and buff with a soft, lint free cloth to get a shiny clean surface that will look like you have just purchased new fittings every time!

Safety Issues and Precautions

Apple cider vinegar is a particularly powerful substance. As we have seen, it has a strong effect on the body, it is strong enough to remove mold and limescale from your home and eradicate nits and fleas from your pets and therefore must be used with caution.

Speak to Your Doctor

Before you use any health supplement, tonic or begin adding anything new to your diet, consult your doctor. Ensure your doctor knows what you'll be taking, how much you plan to take and ask for their professional opinion.

If your doctor is skeptical, don't be surprised, but instead ask if he or she knows of any medical reason why taking apple cider vinegar will do you any actual harm. If they do not have any reason why you shouldn't take it, then they should be happy to give you the benefit of the doubt.

Drug Interactions

One of the most important aspects of seeing a medical professional before taking ACV is to make sure that there are not likely to be any interactions between the apple cider vinegar and any medication you're already taking. If your doctor flags a potential problem, take their advice on whether you need to stay on the medication and leave the ACV until a later date.

There may be drug interactions with medications used to treat diabetes, as well as diuretics, and medications that affect the potassium levels in your body.

Diabetes

While ACV can be used to help people with diabetes, it can alter blood sugar levels and so those with the disease need to keep

> "The main thing is to follow the famous phrase 'Keep calm and carry on', don't let a setback throw out your whole program, if you have a bad day or even a bad week, remember the images of the future you and get back on track as quickly as you can."

Osteoporosis

Experts are not in consensus as to whether ACV is beneficial for those with Osteoporosis or whether it's harmful. So, if you think it might be of benefit, speak to an expert and get some advice on whether ACV is the right choice for you.

Pregnancy and Breastfeeding

There has not been enough research conducted on how apple cider vinegar may affect an unborn child. Nor has there been any extensive investigation into the effect on breastfeeding or whether the ACV is secreted into the breast milk, or indeed what affect it would have on the child if it did.

The best advice during pregnancy is generally to avoid substances when their effects are largely unknown. While ACV may seem like a good choice during pregnancy, you would be best advised to avoid it unless given the green light by a medical professional.

a very close check on their blood sugar levels when taking apple cider vinegar. It is essential you speak to your doctor if you have diabetes and are considering taking ACV. Follow their professional advice as each case is unique.

APPLE CIDER VINEGAR RECIPES

As well as taking apple cider vinegar in water, it can be added to all sorts of recipes to boost your intake or even be the actual focus of the meal itself. You can swap your usual vinegar for ACV and experiment with using it in place of wine in some recipes.

The focus here is on healthy recipes that taste great and incorporate ACV. Remember that ACV on its own probably won't give you the weight-loss results you want, but added to a healthy lifestyle, you will reap many rewards.

In keeping with the natural, health-giving properties of apple cider vinegar, these recipes provide you with valuable nutrition and a satisfying wholesome dish of food.

Perhaps you are struggling to think of any of your usual recipes that could incorporate apple cider vinegar... but there is one staple meal that we all turn to that can be even more nutritious and tasty with the addition of simple ACV... salads.

Salads come in all shapes and with so many ingredients and variations, you could eat salad for the rest of your life and never have the same meal twice!

A healthy, filling salad can be one of the best tools in reaching your weight loss goals, it's for this reason that you'll find some great salad recipes and dressings along with smoothies, main meals, and desserts - which all contain ACV.

BREAKFASTS

SUNNY DAY SMOOTHIE

SERVES 2

INGREDIENTS

- 300ml/10 fl oz Orange juice
- 150ml/5 fl oz pineapple juice
- ⅓ cup desiccated coconut
- ½ banana
- 2 tsp fresh ginger, peeled, and chopped
- 1 tbsp apple cider vinegar
- 4 Ice cubes

METHOD

1. Combine all the ingredients except the ice cubes and blend in a blender for 30 seconds.
2. Add the ice cubes gradually and blend for a further 30 seconds.

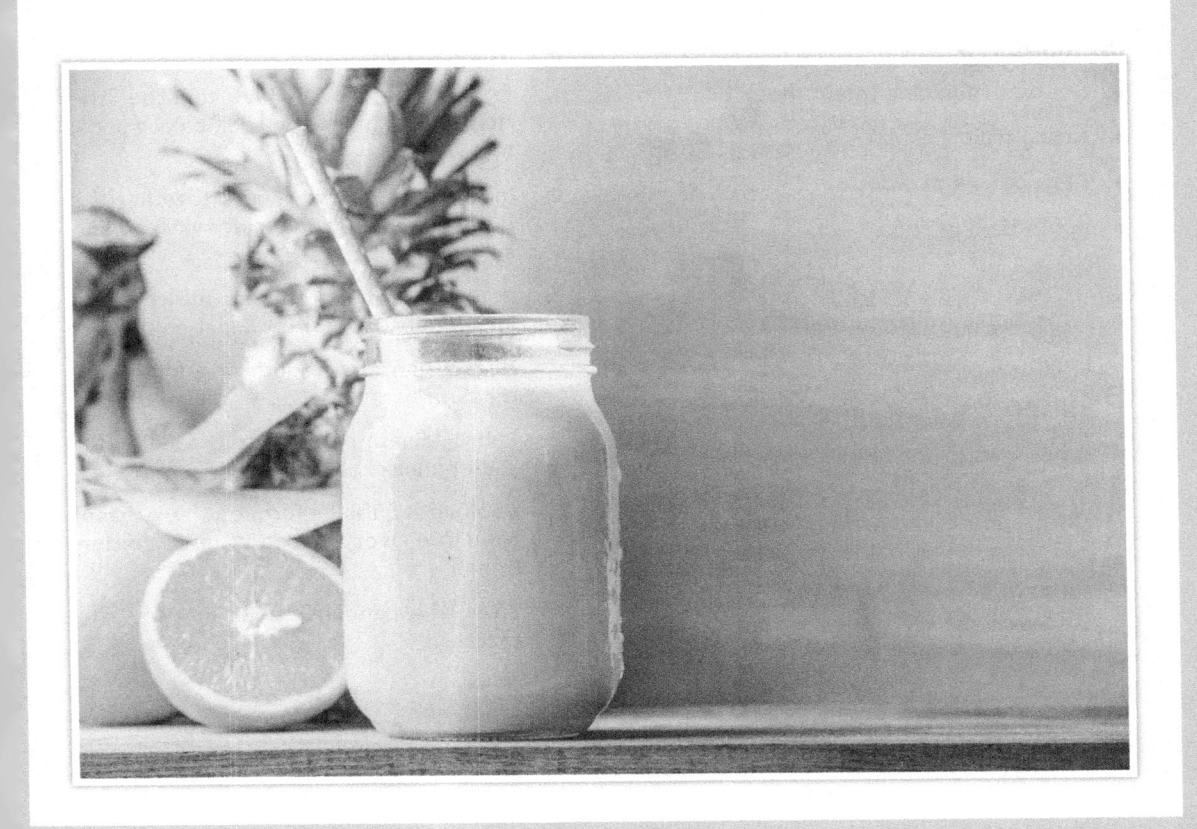

BREAKFASTS | 77

APPLE CIDER VINEGAR SMOOTHIE

SERVES 1

INGREDIENTS

- 1 banana
- 1 cup spinach
- ½ cup unsweetened almond milk
- 1 tbsp apple cider vinegar
- 1 tbsp almond butter
- 1 tbsp honey or maple syrup (optional, for added sweetness)

METHOD

1. Add all the ingredients to a blender.
2. Blend until smooth and creamy.
3. Adjust the sweetness if desired.
4. Pour into a glass and enjoy your ACV-infused smoothie.

APPLE CIDER VINEGAR PANCAKES

SERVES 2

INGREDIENTS

- 1 cup all-purpose (plain) flour
- 1 tbsp fruit sugar
- 1 tsp baking powder
- ½ tsp baking soda
- ¼ tsp salt
- 1 cup buttermilk or low-fat yogurt
- 1 egg
- 1 tbsp apple cider vinegar
- 1 tbsp sunflower oil

METHOD

1. In a mixing bowl, whisk together the flour, sugar, baking powder, baking soda, and salt.
2. In a separate bowl, whisk together the buttermilk, egg, apple cider vinegar, and sunflower oil.
3. Pour the wet ingredients into the dry ingredients and stir until just combined.
4. Heat a non-stick skillet or griddle over medium heat and lightly grease it.
5. Pour ¼ cup of batter onto the skillet for each pancake.
6. Cook until bubbles form on the surface, then flip over and cook until golden brown.
7. Serve the pancakes with your favorite toppings.

OVERNIGHT OATS

SERVES 1

INGREDIENTS

- ½ cup rolled oats
- ½ cup unsweetened almond milk
- ½ cup low fat Greek yogurt
- 1 tbsp chia seeds
- 1 tbsp apple cider vinegar
- 1 tbsp honey or maple syrup
- Optional toppings: diced apples, cinnamon, nuts, or dried fruits

METHOD

1. In a jar or container, combine all the ingredients.
2. Stir well to ensure everything is well mixed.
3. Cover the jar/container and refrigerate overnight.
4. In the morning, give the mixture a good stir.
5. Add your preferred toppings and enjoy your ACV-infused overnight oats.

One of the best uses of the microwave is for preparing this slow release, simple to prepare version of good old porridge. If you have a kitchen area you can use at work, then this is an ideal lunch or mid-afternoon snack.

Generally, you must add a certain amount of milk and then cook on full power for a couple of minutes, but you'll need to check the packet instructions as portion sizes may vary and this will affect the cooking times.

Don't buy the pre-flavored varieties though as these will be packed with sugars and salt. Instead, you can add your own sweeteners and flavorings.

You can try adding fruit sugar, honey, stevia, maple syrup or agave nectar as sweeteners and there are many toppings to add flavor such as figs, raisins, blackcurrants, or dried cherries etc.

If you have a lactose intolerance you can use other forms of milk instead such as goats, rice, oat, soya, or almond milk etc.

FRUIT SALAD WITH YOGURT

SERVES 1

INGREDIENTS

- Assorted fresh fruits and berries of your choice (such as apples, raspberries, grapes, oranges, watermelon etc.)
- 1 tbsp apple cider vinegar
- 1 tbsp honey or agave syrup
- Fresh mint leaves for garnish (optional)
- 2 tbsp fat-free or low-fat unsweetened natural yogurt

METHOD

1. Wash and chop the fruits into bite-sized pieces.
2. In a small bowl, whisk together the apple cider vinegar and honey (or agave syrup) to make the dressing.
3. Drizzle the dressing over the fruit and gently toss to combine.
4. Garnish with fresh mint leaves if desired.
5. Allow the fruit salad to sit for a few minutes before adding the yogurt to let the flavors blend together.

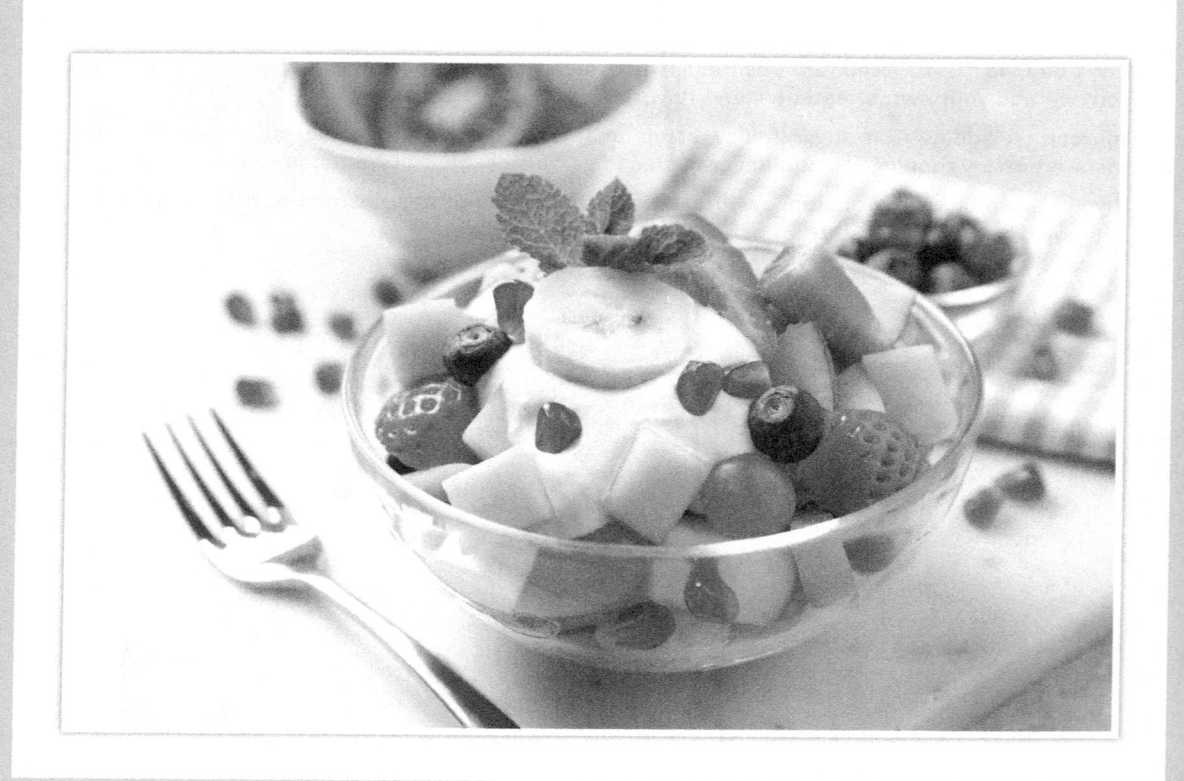

CRUNCHY NUT GRANOLA

INGREDIENTS

- ¼ cup/ 2fl oz maple syrup
- 4 tbsp stevia or agave nectar
- 4 tbsp sunflower oil
- 500g/ 1lb 2oz rolled oats
- 175g/ 6oz seed mix (sunflower, pumpkin, and sesame work well)
- 150g/ 5oz roughly crushed pecans
- 50g/ 2oz raw flaked almonds
- 85g/3oz desiccated coconut (unsweetened)
- 150g/ 5½oz dried fruit (use your favorite)
- 1 tsp ground mixed spice
- 1 tbsp apple cider vinegar
- 1 tsp vanilla extract

METHOD

1. Heat your oven to 160°C /325°F/gas mark 3.
2. Line a large roasting tin with greaseproof paper.
3. Mix the stevia (or agave nectar) with the maple syrup, oil, apple cider vinegar and vanilla extract in a large bowl, to combine fully.
4. Next add the remaining ingredients apart from dried fruit and mix thoroughly.
5. Pour the mix in to the roasting tin and cook for 15 - 20 minutes or until golden brown, turning every 5 minutes.
6. When cooled, add the dried fruit, mix thoroughly and transfer to an airtight container.

This can be served with cow's milk, oat, goat, almond or soya milk or with frozen plain yogurt as a snack at any time of the day.

SPINACH AND MUSHROOM FRITTATA

SERVES 2

No flipping required in this quick-to-prepare, hearty frittata, loaded with antioxidants and terrific flavors.

INGREDIENTS

- 1½ tsp olive oil
- 1 small red potato, cooked, unpeeled, and sliced
- Salt and pepper to taste
- 2 cups fresh baby spinach, roughly chopped
- 1 cup thinly sliced white mushrooms
- 2 large eggs
- 2 large egg whites
- 1 tsp dried thyme
- 2 tsp chopped fresh parsley

METHOD

1. Heat olive oil in a heavy 12-inch flame-proof skillet over medium-high heat. Place a layer of sliced potatoes in a skillet, and sprinkle with pepper. Cook until lightly browned (about 4 minutes), turning slices over once.

2. Add spinach and mushrooms, stir to combine, reduce heat to low, and cook, covered, until spinach leaves have wilted – about 3 minutes.

3. In a medium bowl whisk together the eggs and egg whites, thyme, and parsley. Pour egg mixture into skillet, use a spatula to distribute vegetables evenly, and cook, covered, over medium-low heat until the bottom of the frittata is lightly browned, and eggs are almost set – 6 to 8 minutes.

4. Place the skillet under a broiler or grill, set on a low heat to finish cooking the top of the frittata, for about 2 minutes.

5. 5. Use a metal spatula to loosen the sides and bottom of the frittata, then slide onto a warm platter, and serve immediately.

Variations: Substitute any steamed vegetables for the spinach and mushrooms. On weekends replace the egg whites with whole eggs and stir in ½ cup grated Manchego cheese.

CRANBERRY ZEST

SERVES 2

INGREDIENTS

- 150ml/ 5fl oz cranberry juice
- 4 satsumas/ tangerines or mandarin oranges
- 1 frozen banana (throw a peeled, chopped banana into a freezer bag and freeze overnight)
- 5 large frozen strawberries
- 1 tbsp apple cider vinegar

METHOD

1. In a blender, add in all the ingredients and blend until smooth.
2. Serve immediately or refrigerate until ready to use.

If you've forgotten to freeze the banana or strawberries in advance, don't worry, just use a fresh banana, and add some ice cubes instead.

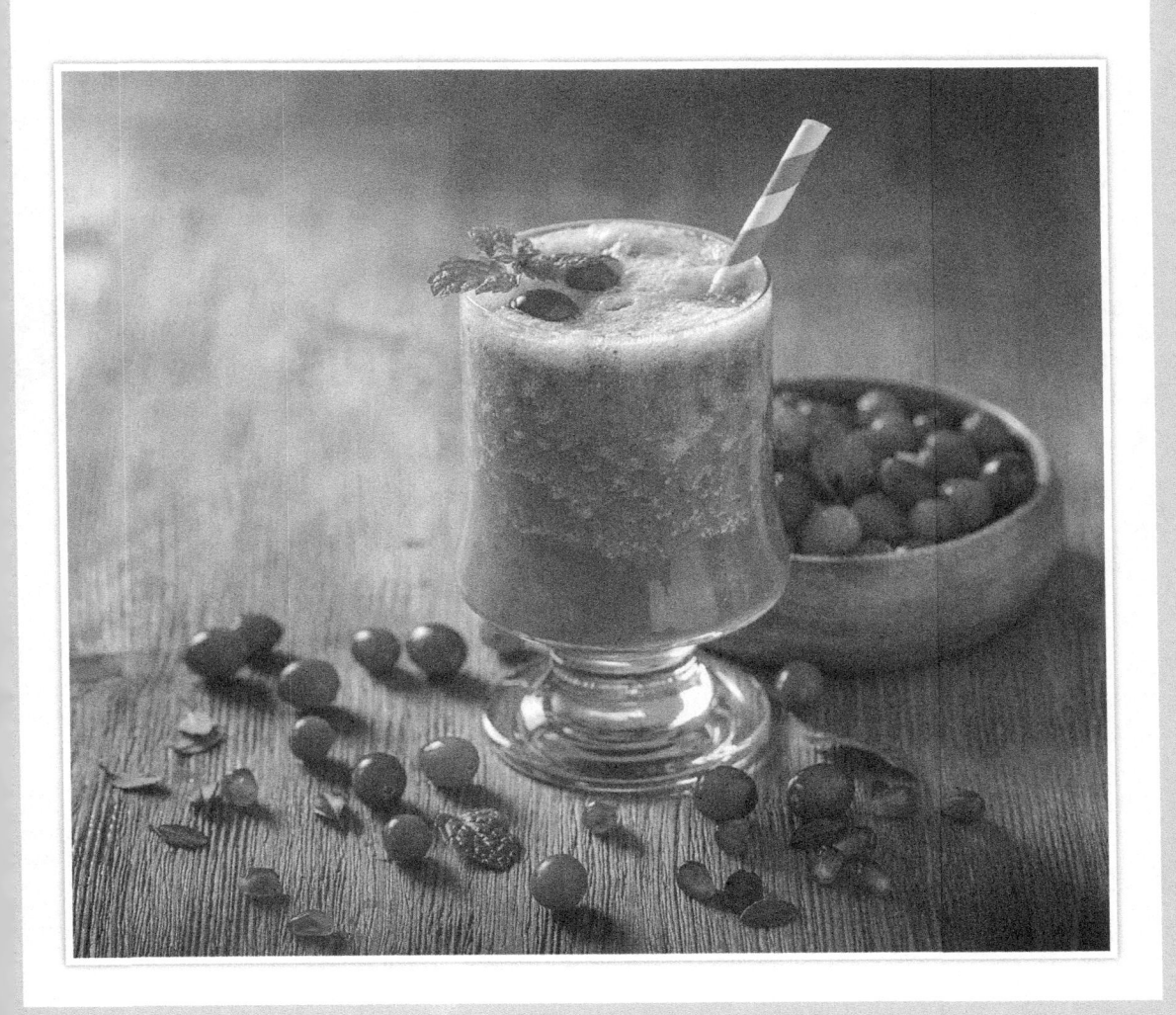

BREAKFASTS | 83

HEALTHY BAKED BEANS WITH POACHED EGGS

SERVES 2

INGREDIENTS

- 400g/16oz can of borlotti beans, drained
- 500g/18oz passata
- 1 garlic clove, peeled and finely chopped
- 1 tsp paprika
- 1 tbsp maple syrup
- 1 tbsp apple cider vinegar
- 1 tbsp Worcestershire sauce
- 1 tbsp olive oil
- 2 free range eggs
- Sea salt and ground black pepper to taste

METHOD

1. Heat the olive oil gently in a large pan then sauté the garlic on a very low heat until transparent, (usually about 2 - 3 minutes) do not allow to burn, so keep stirring.
2. Add the borlotti beans and cook for a further minute or two.
3. Add the passata, paprika, apple cider vinegar, Worcestershire sauce and maple syrup and turn up the heat.
4. Bring to a boil, then lower the heat to a simmer, cover and reduce for 10 minutes.
5. Meanwhile add 2 eggs to a pan of boiling water and poach to your preference.
6. Serve immediately or place any remaining beans in a sealed container to use later.

GINGER KICK GREEN SMOOTHIE

SERVES 1

INGREDIENTS

- ½ inch piece fresh ginger, peeled
- ¼ lemon, peeled
- 1 apple, cored
- 5 stalks kale
- 1 avocado, peeled and sliced
- 1 pinch of sea salt
- 100ml/3½fl oz water

METHOD

1. In a blender, add in all the ingredients and blend until smooth
2. Serve immediately or refrigerate until ready to use.

LUNCHES

INDONESIAN SALAD

SERVES 4

This is an exotic, fruity salad that is perfect for long summer evenings, as an accompaniment to a barbecue or to bring a taste of summer to any occasion. The flavors blend to create an unforgettable taste that is truly impressive.

INGREDIENTS

- 1 tin pineapple chunks
- ½ cucumber, cut into matchsticks
- 175g carrots, peeled and cut into matchsticks
- 1 crisp green eating apple, cored, quartered, and chopped roughly
- 125g bean sprouts

DRESSING

- 1 tbsp crunchy peanut butter, with no added sugar or salt
- 2 tbsp soy sauce
- 1 tbsp olive oil
- 1 tbsp. apple cider vinegar
- Juice of ½ lemon
- Salt and pepper

METHOD

1. Combine all the salad ingredients together.
2. To make the dressing, put the peanut butter in a bowl and gradually whisk in the other ingredients with a fork and season with salt and pepper.
3. Pour the dressing over the salad and toss well to mix. Cover and leave to stand for 30 minutes before serving.

CHICKEN STIR FRY

SERVES 2

INGREDIENTS

- 1 tbsp olive oil
- 1 garlic clove crushed or peeled and finely chopped
- 2 skinless chicken breasts, cut into ½ inch strips (you can use Quorn or Soya chunks instead)
- 1 red pepper, washed, cored, and chopped into 1-inch squares
- 4 large mushrooms, wiped with a damp cloth, stalk removed and thinly sliced
- 1 medium carrot, scrubbed, peeled, and then cut into matchstick sized pieces
- 1 medium onion, peeled and finely chopped
- Handful mangetout, washed and cut into matchstick-sized pieces
- 1 tbsp light soy sauce
- 1 tbsp apple cider vinegar
- 100ml/ 3½fl oz chicken stock

METHOD

1. Heat the olive oil in a wok or large frying pan on a low heat. Add the chicken pieces and cook, turning occasionally until the flesh is slightly browned all over.
2. Add the onion and stir for a few minutes.
3. Next, add the pepper, carrot, mangetout, to the pan and stir-fry for 2 - 3 minutes.
4. Turn down the heat and add the garlic. Cook for a further 2 minutes, stirring constantly.
5. Finally add the chicken stock and light soy sauce. Cook on a medium heat setting until the chicken and vegetables are thoroughly cooked.
6. Serve with boiled brown rice, buckwheat, or pearl barley.

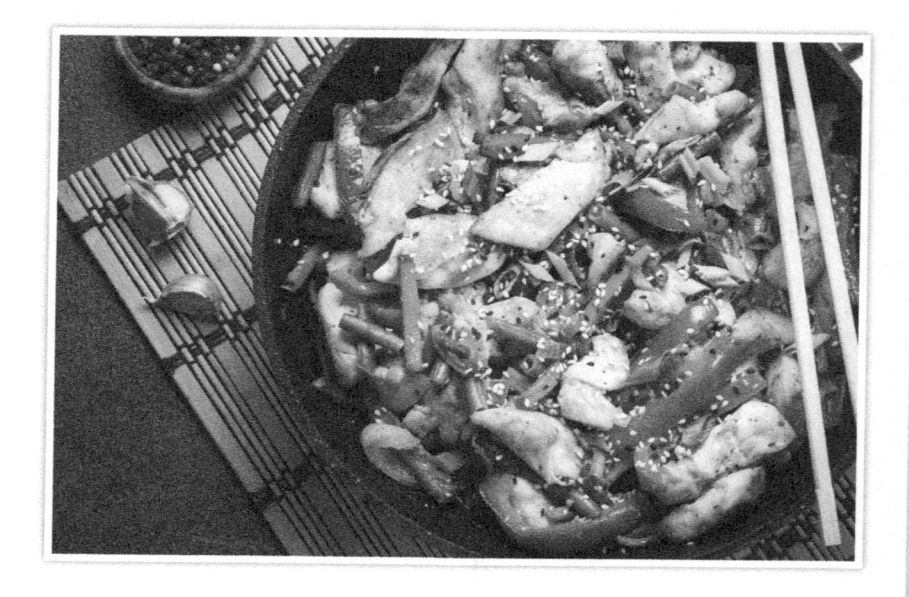

NEW POTATO SALAD

SERVES 4-6

INGREDIENTS

- 1lb/450g small new potatoes, cooked
- 1 bunch watercress, washed and finely chopped
- 1 garlic clove, crushed
- 1oz/25g walnuts, finely chopped
- 5oz/150g low-fat natural yogurt
- Salt and pepper to taste
- 1 tbsp apple cider vinegar
- 1 tsp maple syrup

METHOD

1. Drain potatoes and leave until cold then cut into halves.
2. Mix together watercress, garlic, and walnuts. Add yogurt, apple cider vinegar, maple syrup, season and mix thoroughly.
3. Add potatoes and stir ensuring that everything is well mixed, refrigerate for about 30 minutes before serving.

CHICKEN AND BACON SALAD

SERVES 2

INGREDIENTS

- 2 chicken breasts, skin removed
- 4 slices back bacon
- Salad vegetables to taste
- 8 new potatoes, cooked and halved

DRESSING

- 1 tbsp clear honey
- 1 tbsp apple cider vinegar
- 1 tbsp olive oil
- 1 tsp wholegrain mustard
- Salt and pepper

METHOD

1. Combine dressing ingredients thoroughly.
2. Marinate chicken in the dressing for one hour.
3. Place on a baking tray making sure chicken is well coated.
4. Bake in oven for about 20 minutes or until juices run clear.
5. Allow to cool slightly and then cut into 4 chunks.
6. Meanwhile grill the bacon until crispy, then blot with kitchen paper and remove all visible fat before cutting into strips.
7. Prepare salad vegetables and arrange in serving bowl.
8. Place chicken, bacon, and potatoes on top.

LUNCHES | 87

APPLE CIDER VINEGAR-MARINATED PORK CHOPS

SERVES 2

The combination of pork and apple is an absolute cookery classic. The flavors work so well together!

Next time you cook pork, set aside the apple sauce, and aim instead to make use of apple cider vinegar to boost the flavor and succulence of the meat to create a truly unforgettable meal.

INGREDIENTS

- 1 cup apple cider vinegar
- ¼ cup olive oil
- 4 cloves, minced garlic
- 3 – 4 sprigs rosemary
- 3 – 4 bay leaves
- 1 tbsp brown sugar
- 4 pork chops, raw (alternatively use pork pieces)

METHOD

1. Whisk together the ingredients for the marinade.
2. Place the pork chops in the marinade and make sure they are fully coated.
3. Cover and refrigerate for an hour before cooking.
4. Broil/grill the pork chops on a medium heat or for a fantastic smoky flavor, place on the barbecue.
5. Ensure the pork is completely cooked through before serving with baby new potatoes and fresh spring greens. A slice of apple on top of each pork chop adds a nice touch

APPLE AND BUTTERNUT SQUASH SOUP

SERVES 4

This is a lovely, sweet soup, and the addition of the vinegar gives it the edge it needs to prevent it from being too sweet. The blend of flavors makes for a truly memorable meal – you can experiment with the recipe by adding some of your favorite herbs and spices to create a unique dish.

INGREDIENTS

- 1 medium butternut squash, cubed
- 2 apples, peeled, cored, and sliced
- 1 large, sweet potato, cubed
- 1 onion, finely chopped
- 4 – 5 cloves garlic, finely chopped
- 3 tbsp softened butter (you can use softened coconut butter if you prefer)
- 3 cups vegetable stock
- 1 cup coconut milk
- 3 tbsp apple cider vinegar
- 1 tsp ground mixed herbs
- 1 tsp ground cumin
- ½ tsp salt
- Black pepper – to taste

METHOD

1. Place a large pan on the hob; add the butter, onions, cumin and garlic and sauté over a medium heat until the onions are soft- but be careful not to burn the garlic.
2. Add the butternut squash, apple and the sweet potato and stir over the medium heat for a few minutes.
3. Add the stock, apple cider vinegar, and the herbs.
4. Simmer for an hour or until the potato, apple and squash are soft.
5. Using a mixer or food processor, blend the soup until it is smooth and then return it to the pan.
6. Reheat the soup until simmering gently, then remove from the heat.
7. Stir in the coconut milk just before serving the soup and add pepper to taste.

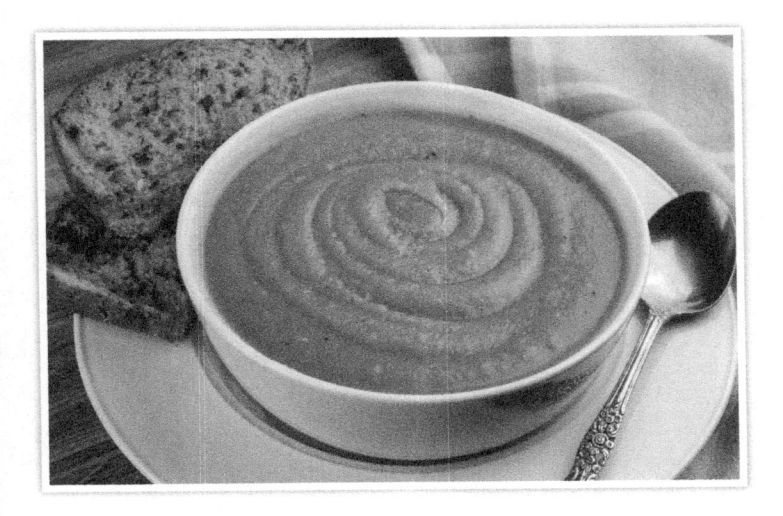

LUNCHES | 89

GRILLED VEGETABLE SALAD

SERVES 4

INGREDIENTS

- 1 red pepper
- 1 green pepper
- 350g courgettes
- 6 whole garlic cloves
- 1 bunch of asparagus
- Olive oil, for brushing
- Handful cherry tomatoes
- Chopped herbs – e.g., basil, marjoram, thyme, parsley, or chives

DRESSING

- 2 tsp balsamic vinegar
- 1 tsp thin honey or natural maple syrup
- ½ tsp Dijon mustard
- 1 tbsp olive oil
- 1 tbsp apple cider vinegar
- Salt and pepper

METHOD

1. Halve the peppers and remove the seeds and cores. Cut each half into four.
2. Thickly slice the courgettes on the diagonal. Remove the loose, papery outer skins from the garlic cloves but leave the inner skins attached.
3. Steam the asparagus until tender, drain and arrange on a serving plate.
4. Brush the peppers, courgette and garlic with oil and cook under a hot grill until flecked with brown. Turn the vegetables over and cook on the other side. Once cooled, arrange on the plate with asparagus. Halve the tomatoes and scatter over the vegetables.
5. To make the dressing, put the vinegar, honey, apple cider vinegar and mustard into a small bowl and whisk together with a fork until well-blended. Gradually whisk in the oil to make a very thick dressing. Season with salt and pepper.
6. Just before serving, drizzle the dressing over the vegetables and sprinkle with the chopped herbs.

SPANISH PRAWNS AND MIXED LEAF SALAD

SERVES 2

For the prawns and sauce

INGREDIENTS

- 200g raw or frozen uncooked prawns
- ⅓ cup of apple juice
- 1 tbsp apple cider vinegar
- Juice of ½ lemon
- 3 big cloves of garlic finely minced
- 2 tsp paprika
- ½ tsp turmeric
- ½ tsp ground cumin
- ¼ tsp chipotle flakes
- 1 tsp smoked paprika
- 1 tsp vegetable stock powder or fish stock
- 1 tsp fruit sugar or maple syrup
- 1 tbsp olive oil

MIXED LEAF SALAD DRESSING

- 2 cups mixed leaves
- 2 tsp balsamic vinegar
- 1 tsp runny honey
- 1/2 tsp Dijon mustard
- 1 tbsp olive oil
- 1 tbsp apple cider vinegar
- Salt and pepper

METHOD

1. Add the minced garlic to a pan with a little oil and (bring gently up to heat) cook over a gentle heat, making sure not to burn the garlic.
2. Next add the vegetable or fish stock and the apple juice along with the rest of the ingredients for the prawn recipe- but not the prawns themselves. Reduce over a gentle heat until the sauce thickens.
3. In a separate pan, cook the raw prawns on a medium heat for a couple of minutes, turning regularly until they turn a uniform shade of pink.
4. Then add them to the prawn sauce and cook for a further 5 minutes on a low heat.
5. To make the dressing for the mixed leaf salad, put the vinegar, honey, apple cider vinegar and mustard into a small bowl and whisk together with a fork until well blended. Gradually whisk in the olive oil to make a thicker dressing. Season with salt and pepper.
6. Just before serving, drizzle the dressing over the mixed leaves.

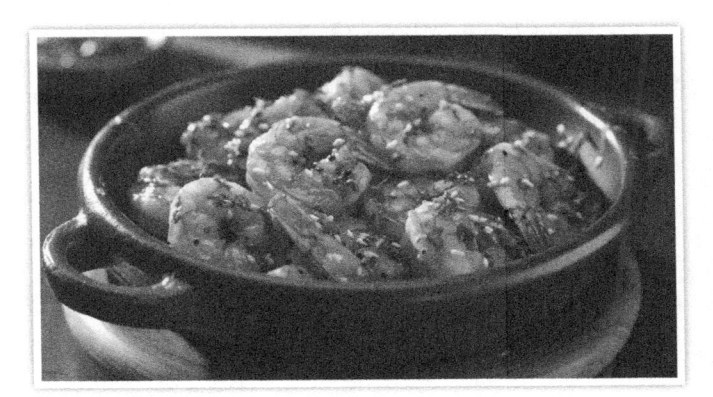

LUNCHES

TOMATO, ROCKET, AND SUGAR SNAP PEA SALAD

SERVES 4

This is such a simple idea for a salad; you won't believe how well the flavors work together. Try to choose the freshest, sweetest cherry tomatoes you can find to really get the most out of this delicious meal.

INGREDIENTS

- 175g sugar snap peas
- 125g rocket
- 225g cherry tomatoes, halved

DRESSING

- 1 tbsp olive oil
- 1 tbsp apple cider vinegar
- ½ tsp wholegrain mustard
- Salt and pepper

METHOD

1. Add the peas to boiling water and simmer for 4 – 5 minutes. Drain and refresh in cold water. Pat dry on kitchen paper.
2. Mix the rocket, tomatoes, and peas together.
3. Whisk all the dressing ingredients together, pour over the salad, tossing to coat well.
4. Serve immediately.

FRENCH ONION SOUP

SERVES 4

INGREDIENTS

- 1lb/ 700g onions, peeled and chopped
- 2 cloves garlic, peeled and finely chopped
- 1 tsp fruit sugar or brown sugar
- ½ tbsp butter or coconut butter
- 1 large potato, peeled and diced
- 2 tsp olive oil
- 1½ pints vegetable stock
- 1 tbsp apple cider vinegar
- Black pepper

METHOD

1. Add butter and olive oil to a saucepan on a high heat and add onions and sugar. Cook for about 5 – 10 minutes or until caramelised, stirring continuously.
2. Turn the heat down to a simmer and add garlic and potato. Continue to cook with the pan covered for about 20 minutes.
3. Add the vegetable stock, bring to the boil, then simmer uncovered for about 20 minutes to reduce.
4. Blend leaving a little texture and serve with French bread or warm wholemeal bread torn into chunks.

DINNERS

SEARED STEAK WITH MUSHROOMS

SERVES 1

Lean beef combined with earthy mushrooms in this easy dish prepared with a simple and quick red wine sauce.

INGREDIENTS

- 2 tsp olive oil
- 2 cups sliced mushrooms (any variety will do)
- Salt and pepper to taste
- 2 tsp chopped fresh thyme or 1 tsp dried thyme
- 14 oz. sirloin or tenderloin beef steak
- 1 tbsp red wine
- 1 tbsp apple cider vinegar

METHOD

1. Heat 1 tsp of oil in a large non-stick skillet over medium-high heat. Add mushrooms, season with salt and pepper and cook, stirring occasionally, until softened and golden. This takes about 6 minutes. Add thyme and cook 1 minute more. Set aside, keeping warm.

2. Heat remaining oil in a large heavy skillet over medium-high heat. Season both sides of steaks with salt and pepper, and add to skillet, cooking to desired taste - about 4 minutes per side for medium-rare. Remove steak from the skillet and set aside to rest. Meanwhile pour wine and apple cider vinegar into hot skillet and bring to a simmer for a couple of minutes, then remove from heat.

3. To serve, place steak in middle of plate, spoon sauce over and top with the mushrooms.

Variations: On weekends select rib eye or porterhouse.

VEGAN BURRITOS

SERVES 4

INGREDIENTS

- 4 large wholemeal tortilla wraps
- Washed spinach leaves, shredded
- 1 avocado, thinly sliced or mashed into a paste
- Chilli sauce, to serve

FOR THE BLACK BEANS:

- 1 tbsp olive oil
- 1 garlic clove, finely chopped or minced
- 1 tbsp apple cider vinegar
- 1 tsp dried chipotle or ancho chilli flakes
- 400g can chopped tomatoes
- 400g black beans, drained
- 1 bunch cilantro, chopped

FOR THE LIME AND RED ONION RICE:

- 250g wholegrain rice, cooked and drained
- 1 lime, juiced
- ½ red onion, very finely chopped
- 50g pistachio nuts, roughly chopped

METHOD

1. To make the beans, heat the oil in a pan and fry the garlic for a minute, then stir in the chipotle flakes and the apple cider vinegar. Tip in the tomatoes, stir and bring to a simmer until the sauce thickens, season with salt. Simmer until thick, add the beans and cook briefly (make sure any water gets cooked off), then stir in the cilantro.

2. If you are using cold cooked rice, then warm it through, stir in the lime juice, red onion and nuts and season well or cook rice as per packet instructions.

3. Lay out the tortillas and sprinkle over some spinach. Add some avocado slices and some rice, then top with the bean mix. Add a shake of hot sauce, if you like. Roll the bottom up, then fold the sides in to stop the filling falling out as you roll. Wrap tightly in foil and cut in half.

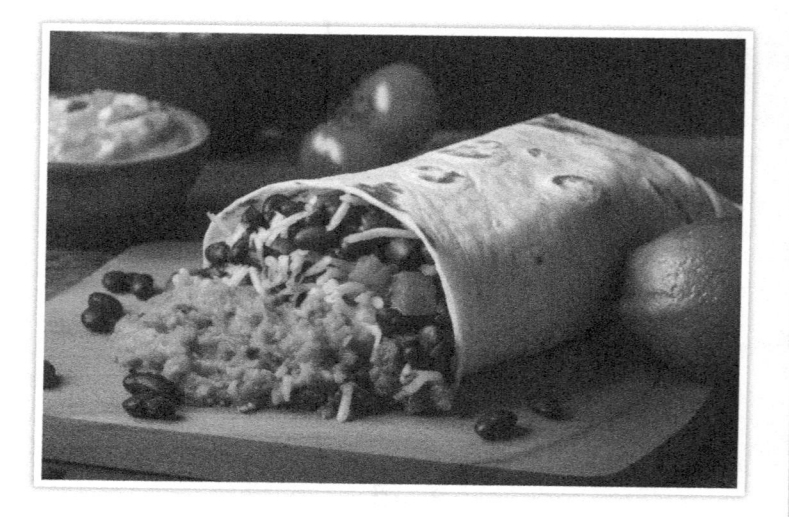

BEEF STIR FRY

Serves 2

INGREDIENTS

- 1 tbsp olive oil
- 1 garlic clove crushed or peeled and finely chopped
- 12 ounces of lean beef
- 1 red pepper, washed, cored, and chopped in to 1-inch squares
- 4 large mushrooms, wiped with a damp cloth, stalk removed and thinly sliced
- 1 medium carrot, scrubbed, peeled, and then cut into matchstick-sized pieces
- 1 medium onion, peeled and finely chopped
- 1 tbsp light soy sauce
- 1 tbsp apple cider vinegar
- ½ cup beef stock

METHOD

1. Heat the olive oil in a wok or large frying pan over a low heat.
2. Add the beef pieces and cook, turning occasionally, until it's lightly browned all over. Add the onion and stir for a few minutes.
3. Next, add the pepper and carrot to the pan and stir-fry for 2 - 3 minutes.
4. Turn down the heat and add the garlic. Cook for 2 minutes, stirring constantly.
5. Finally add the beef stock, apple cider vinegar and light soy sauce and cook on a medium heat setting until the beef and vegetables are thoroughly cooked.
6. Serve with your choice of a mixed salad or freshly steamed vegetables and enjoy.

PRAWN CURRY

SERVES 2

INGREDIENTS

- 1 medium onion, peeled and finely chopped
- 2 cloves of garlic, peeled and finely chopped
- 500g/17oz tomato passata (sieved tomatoes, but canned chopped tomatoes will do)
- 50g/1.5oz ground almonds
- 1 rounded tbsp Madras or Korma (no cream added) curry paste (these are the pastes made from the spices and herbs etc. for the base of the curry, NOT a pre-brought sauce)
- 2 tsp paprika
- 2 tsp olive oil
- 100ml/3fl oz fish or vegetable stock
- 200g cooked king prawns
- Good handful of fresh cilantro, washed thoroughly and finely chopped (some reserved for the garnish)
- Scallions (green onions), washed thoroughly and chopped into small pieces
- 1 tbsp apple cider vinegar
- Juice of 1 lime (some reserved for the garnish)

METHOD

1. Heat the olive oil in a large pan and add the chopped onion.
2. Cook on a medium to low heat for 5 minutes or until the onion takes on a clear, opaque appearance.
3. Turn down the heat and add the chopped garlic, cook for a further 2 - 3 minutes, stirring all the time.
4. Then add the vegetable or fish stock and the curry paste, then turn up the heat for 5 minutes.
5. Next add the passata, lime juice, apple cider vinegar, paprika and chopped cilantro, and simmer to reduce for around 15 minutes.
6. Then add the ground almonds and prawns before seasoning to taste with salt and black pepper.
7. Cook for a further 5 minutes, then garnish with a squeeze of lime juice, some of the chopped cilantro and the scallions.
8. Serve and enjoy.

Serve with your choice of brown rice, buckwheat, or pearl barley. Follow the on-packet cooking instructions for these.

QUICK THAI FISHCAKES

SERVES 2

INGREDIENTS

- 250g/8 oz salmon fillets (skinned and boned)
- 2 tbsp fish sauce (no sugar added)
- 1 tbsp Thai red curry paste
- ½ red onion
- 1 tbsp fresh cilantro (washed and chopped)
- 1 egg white
- Juice and zest of 1 lime
- 1 tbsp olive oil

METHOD

1. Place all the ingredients into a food processor and blend until you have a smooth mixture.
2. Turn out into a mixing bowl.
3. Lightly wet your hands and take the mixture and make in to 4 - 5cm/2-inch rounds about 1cm/½ inch thick.
4. Heat the olive oil in a large non-stick frying pan and cook for 2 - 3 minutes on each side until lightly golden brown.
5. These can be eaten straight away or wrapped in foil and eaten throughout the day as a great protein packed snack.

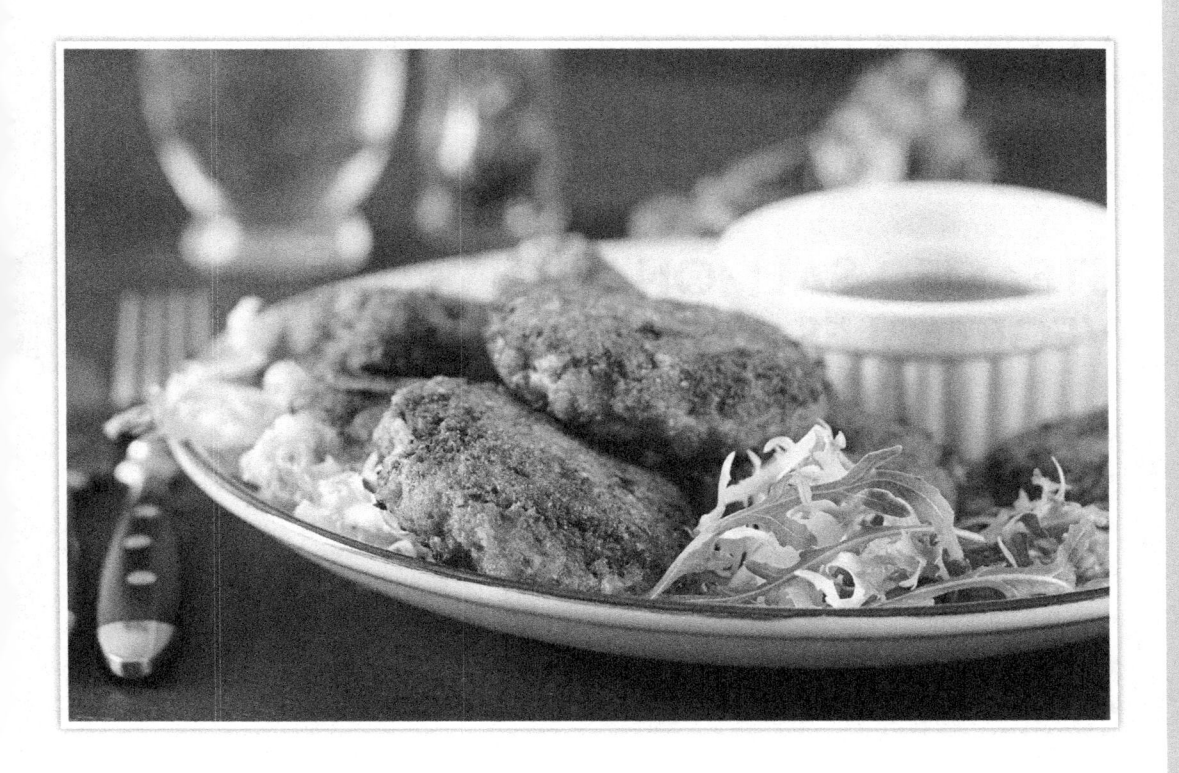

CHICKEN STRIPS WITH SATAY SAUCE

SERVES 1

INGREDIENTS FOR THE CHICKEN

- 1 chicken breast
- 2 tsp olive oil
- 1 tbsp low-salt soy sauce
- Squeeze of fresh lime juice (approx. ½ tbsp)

INGREDIENTS FOR THE PEANUT SAUCE

- 1 tbsp smooth peanut butter (no added sugar)
- 1 tbsp low salt soy sauce
- 1 tbsp apple cider vinegar
- 1 tbsp fresh lime juice
- 1 tsp stevia or agave nectar
- Sprinkling of chopped chives
- Sprinkling of dried garlic powder
- Sprinkling of chili flakes

METHOD

1. Cut the chicken in to strips and flatten them down with a meat mallet, a rolling pin, or the heel of your hand.
2. Place in a container with the soy sauce and olive oil and shake or mix so the chicken gets coated and leave to marinade for 30 minutes.
3. Combine all the peanut sauce ingredients together and whisk with a fork and transfer to a small bowl or container.
4. Heat a griddle pan over a medium heat and place the chicken strips on it.
5. Cook the chicken until it's a golden-brown color, which should take 2 – 3 minutes on each side.
6. 5. Serve the chicken strips with the peanut dipping sauce.

STEAMED SALMON WITH VEGETABLES AND HERBS

SERVES 2

INGREDIENTS

- 2 thinly sliced medium zucchini
- 1 cup cherry tomatoes, cut in half
- 3 tbsp torn sweet basil leaves
- 4 tsp olive oil
- 1 tsp lemon juice
- 1 tbsp apple cider vinegar
- ¼ tsp salt
- 8 tsp chicken stock
- 4 boneless, skinless salmon fillets

METHOD

1. Heat oven to 450°F (230°C).
2. Toss the zucchini, tomatoes and basil leaves with the olive oil, apple cider vinegar and lemon juice.
3. Divide mixture evenly among four foil pouches, topping with salmon and two teaspoons of stock per pouch to help generate steam for moist cooking.
4. Season with salt and pepper to taste and fold packets to seal.
5. Place foil pouches on a baking sheet and bake for about 20 minutes.

BEAN GOULASH

SERVES 2

INGREDIENTS

- 1 red pepper, ½ yellow and ½ green pepper
- 1 medium sized onion
- 400g/14 oz tin drained kidney beans (no sugar/salt added)
- Cup of mushrooms
- 300ml/¾ pint/9 fl oz vegetable stock
- 1 tbsp tomato puree
- 1 tsp mixed herb
- 3 tsp paprika
- 1 clove of garlic
- 1 tbsp apple cider vinegar
- Freshly ground black pepper
- 2 tsp olive oil

METHOD

1. Finely chop onion and garlic, dice peppers and slice mushrooms.
2. Heat oil in saucepan and sauté onion and garlic until onions are transparent.
3. Add paprika and cook for 1 minute, stirring continuously.
4. Add mushrooms and peppers and cook for a further minute, continue stirring.
5. Add remaining ingredients and simmer uncovered until peppers become tender, and sauce thickens.
6. Serve with brown rice, couscous, or noodles.

Diced chicken can be added to this if preferred.

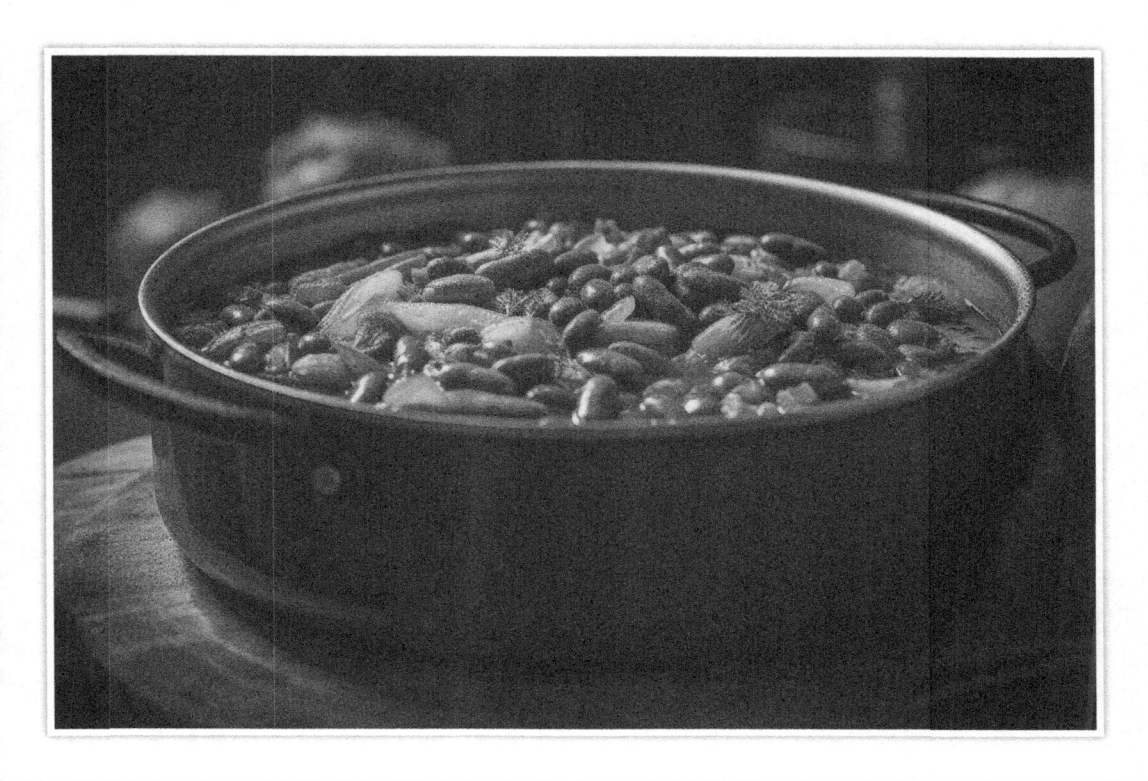

DINNERS

HALIBUT STEW WITH CANNELLINI BEANS

Full of marvelous flavor and color from the addition of a pinch of saffron, this hearty Mediterranean-style stew can also be made with other firm fleshed fish or even shrimp.

INGREDIENTS

- 1 tbsp olive oil
- 1 medium onion, diced
- 1 medium celery stalk, diced
- 1 medium carrot, diced
- 4 garlic cloves, finely chopped
- 1½ cups diced tomatoes (fresh or tinned) with juice
- 1½ cups low-sodium chicken or fish stock
- 1 tbsp apple cider vinegar
- ½ cup water
- Pinch saffron threads
- 400g tin (15-ounce) cannellini beans, drained and rinsed
- 450g (1lb) halibut fillets, cut into chunks
- Salt and pepper to taste
- 1 tbsp chopped fresh parsley

METHOD

1. Heat oil in a large heavy-bottomed pot over medium heat. Add onion, celery, and carrots and cook, stirring occasionally, until softened, about 6 minutes. Add garlic and cook for a further minute.

2. Stir in the tomatoes, stock, water, and saffron. Increase heat to high and bring to a boil. Reduce heat to medium-low and simmer, stirring occasionally, for 5 minutes.

3. Add beans and fish and simmer, covered, until halibut is opaque, and stew is piping hot - about 5 minutes. Season with pepper and serve sprinkled with fresh parsley.

Variations: Substitute chickpeas, butter beans, or a combination of beans for the cannellini beans and on weekends or for a slightly more indulgent touch, add 1 cup cooked diced potatoes.

MEDITERRANEAN BURGER

SERVES 1

Lean ground beef is enhanced with the flavors of the Mediterranean by adding garlic, sundried tomatoes, and fresh herbs. Ground flaxseeds add fiber and moisture.

INGREDIENTS

- 115g (4 oz) lean minced beef
- Salt and pepper to taste
- 1 garlic clove, minced
- 1 tbsp chopped sundried tomatoes or 1 tsp sundried tomato paste
- 1 tbsp ground flaxseeds
- 1 tsp each chopped fresh basil and parsley
- 1 tbsp apple cider vinegar
- ½ tbsp balsamic vinegar

FOR SAUCE:

- Juice of ½ lemon
- 1 tsp olive oil
- 1 tsp English or Dijon mustard
- Pinch dried oregano

METHOD

1. In a small bowl mix together the beef, salt, pepper, garlic, tomatoes, flaxseeds, herbs, balsamic vinegar, and apple cider vinegar. Shape into a burger and set aside.

2. In another small bowl whisk together the lemon juice, olive, oil, mustard, and oregano.

3. Heat a medium nonstick skillet over high heat and brown the burger on both sides until a crust forms, usually around 2 - 3 minutes per side. Cover, reduce the heat to low, and continue to cook to desired taste - a further 5 minutes for medium well done.

4. Transfer the burger to a serving plate and add the sauce mixture to the hot skillet. Stir well and pour over the burger. Serve immediately.

Variations: Make Greek style by replacing beef with minced lamb and basil with fresh mint. On weekends add 2 Tablespoons of crumbled feta cheese for an extra treat.

HEALTHY SNACKS

HOME MADE HUMMUS

SERVES 3-4

This is a tasty little snack, full of protein and bags of flavor. The hummus is easy and quick to make plus you don't need to have any cooking skills. It'll last for 2 or 3 days if it's in a sealed container in your refrigerator.

The wonderful thing about dips is the foods that you eat them with. Try carrot sticks, sliced peppers, baby corn, mangetout, baby tomatoes, broccoli florets... Almost any vegetable you can think of will go very well with this dip. Here's the recipe...

INGREDIENTS

- 200g/7oz canned chickpeas in brine
- 1 garlic clove, peeled and finely chopped
- 1 tbsp freshly squeezed lemon juice
- 1 tbsp apple cider vinegar
- ¼ tsp ground cumin
- Pinch of sea salt
- 1 tsp tahini (sesame seed paste) or unsweetened peanut butter optional
- Water as needed
- 2 tbsp good quality olive oil
- Dusting of smoked paprika

METHOD

1. Place the chickpeas in a colander and rinse in fresh, clean running water, then drain.
2. In a food processor or blender add all the ingredients and blitz for a minute or until the desired consistency is reached.
3. Taste the mixture and add more lemon juice, salt or cumin if needed. (Adjust this to your own taste)
4. To serve, drizzle with a little olive oil and lemon juice and a dusting of paprika.

MEXICAN GUACAMOLE

SERVES 2

INGREDIENTS

- ½ peeled and finely chopped red onion
- 1 ripe avocado, peeled, chopped
- 1 garlic clove, peeled and finely chopped
- ¼ red chili, seeded and finely chopped
- 1 tbsp finely chopped fresh cilantro
- 1 tsp lemon or lime juice
- 1 tbsp apple cider vinegar
- Sea salt to taste
- 2 roughly chopped baby tomatoes
- Paprika to garnish

METHOD

1. Place all the ingredients - apart from the chopped tomatoes - into a blender and mix until combined but not completely smooth.
2. Transfer to a serving bowl and quickly mix in the roughly chopped tomatoes.
3. Serve with vegetable crudités.

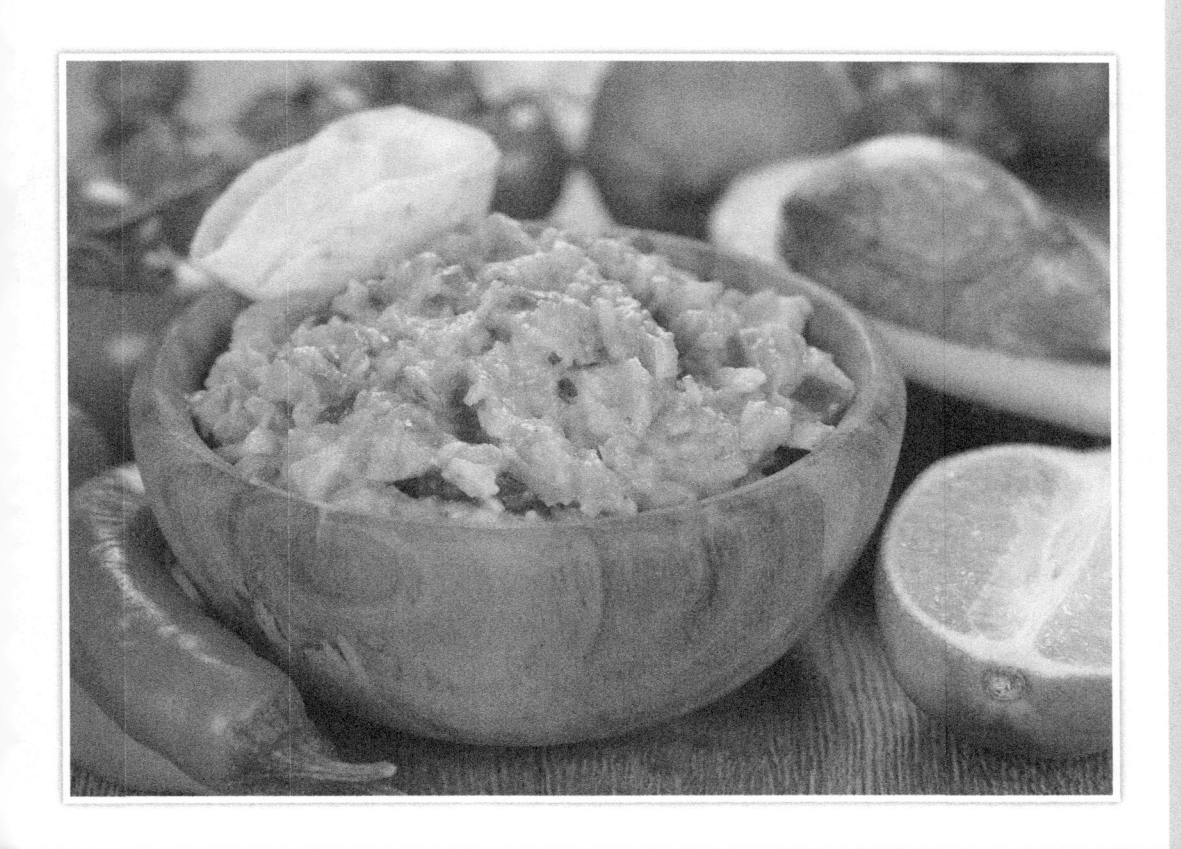

Healthy Snacks | 103

HOMEMADE SLAW

SERVES 4

INGREDIENTS

- ¼ red or white cabbage, finely chopped
- ¼ bulb fennel, peeled and grated
- ½ stick celery, finely chopped
- 1 apple, scrubbed and grated, then tossed in lemon juice to stop discoloration
- 1 carrot, peeled and grated
- 4 walnuts, roughly chopped
- Juice from ½ lemon

DRESSING INGREDIENTS

- 1 tbsp apple cider vinegar
- 2 tsp Dijon mustard
- 2 tsp runny honey
- 2 tsp olive oil
- Pinch of salt

METHOD

1. Toss all the ingredients together - apart from the walnuts- in a large salad bowl.
2. Heat a dry frying pan on a high heat and throw in the chopped walnuts. Cook for 2 minutes.
3. Mix all the dressing ingredients together in a small bowl and whisk until thoroughly combined.
4. Add the walnuts and dressing to the other ingredients and mix to coat evenly.
5. Serve and enjoy.

ONION AND TOMATO SALSA

SERVES 2

INGREDIENTS

- 1 onion, peeled and chopped
- 3 ripe tomatoes, washed, cores removed and chopped
- 1 tsp balsamic vinegar
- 1 tbsp apple cider vinegar
- The juice and zest of ½ lemon (use an unwaxed lemon for this)
- 1 tbsp washed and finely chopped cilantro
- 2 tsp olive oil
- Pinch of sea salt to taste
- Black pepper

METHOD

Combine all ingredients together in a bowl and serve with dry crackers, a poppadum or oven baked flat breads or wraps.

SPICED WHOLE-GRAIN BANANA BREAD

SERVES 4

INGREDIENTS

- 1½ cups whole wheat flour
- ½ cup rolled oats
- ¼ cup ground flax
- 2 tsp baking powder
- 1 tsp cinnamon
- ½ tsp Chinese five spice
- ½ tsp salt
- 3 very ripe bananas, mashed
- 6 tbsp agave syrup
- 1 tbsp apple cider vinegar
- ¾ cup milk or milk substitute
- 4 egg whites
- 1 tsp vanilla extract
- ¾ cup chopped pecans, toasted

METHOD

1. Preheat oven to 350°F (175°C). Grease a standard loaf pan and dust the inside lightly with flour.
2. In a large bowl, blend flour, oats, flax, baking powder, baking soda, cinnamon, and salt, and set aside.
3. Meanwhile, beat egg whites and agave syrup until the mixture forms soft peaks. Gently fold in the milk, bananas and vanilla and mix gently.
4. Pour the wet ingredients into the dry ingredients and combine just until blended. Add pecans and stir until combined.
5. Pour mixture into loaf pan and bake 40 - 50 minutes, until an inserted toothpick comes out clean.

BAKED SPICED PEARS

SERVES 2

INGREDIENTS

- 2 ripe pears
- 2 tbsp coconut or granulated sugar
- 1 tbsp apple cider vinegar
- ¼ tsp ground cinnamon
- ¼ tsp ground cardamom
- 8 ounces low-fat Greek yogurt
- 2 tbsp agave nectar or maple syrup

METHOD

1. Preheat the oven to 350°F (175°C).
2. Peel, halve and core the pears. Place them cut side down in a rectangular baking pan with just enough water to cover the bottom of the pan.
3. Combine the sugar and spices and sprinkle half of the mixture over the pears.
4. Bake the pears for 5 minutes in the preheated oven.
5. Turn the pear halves over, sprinkle with the remaining sugar-spice mixture and continue to bake for another 5 minutes.
6. When pears are fork-tender, remove them from the oven.
7. Meanwhile, mix the yogurt and agave nectar together.
8. Serve pears topped with the sweetened low fat Greek yogurt.

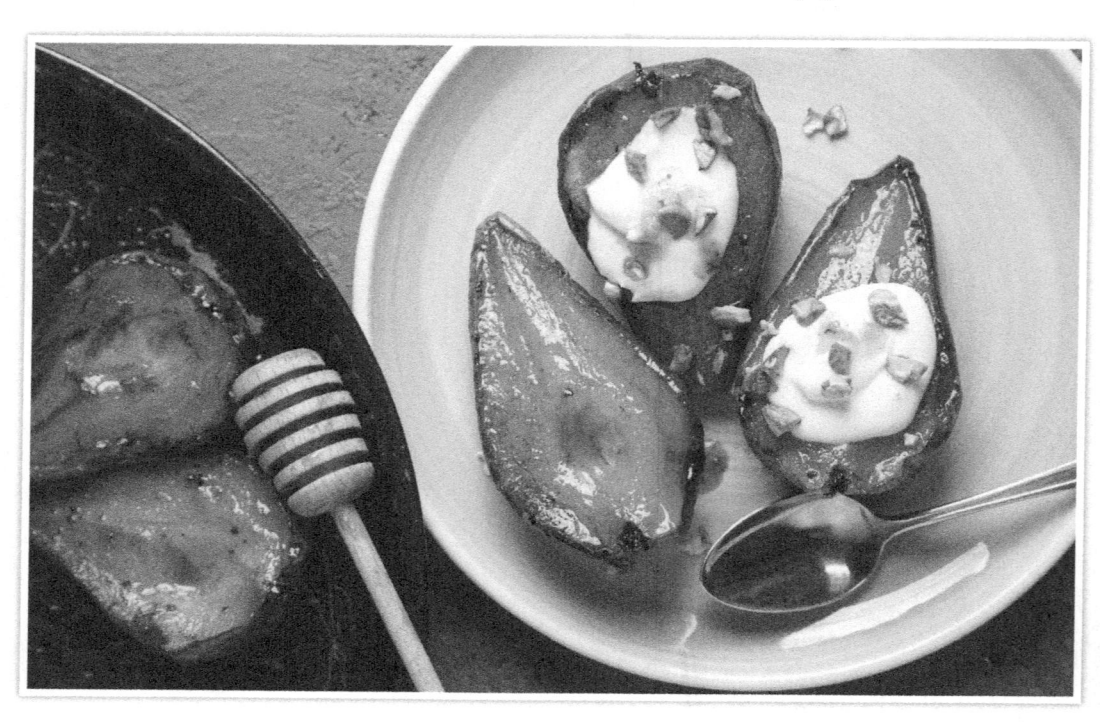

LOW-FAT APPLE CIDER VINEGAR SORBET

SERVES 2

INGREDIENTS

- 2 cups unsweetened apple juice
- ¼ cup apple cider vinegar
- ¼ cup honey or agave syrup
- 1 tbsp lemon juice

INSTRUCTIONS

1. Whisk together the apple juice, apple cider vinegar, honey (or agave syrup), and lemon juice in a large bowl until well combined.
2. Pour the mixture into an ice cream maker and churn according to the manufacturer's instructions.
3. Once the sorbet reaches a slushy consistency, transfer it to a lidded container and freeze for at least 2 - 3 hours to firm up.
4. Serve the low-fat apple cider vinegar sorbet in bowls or cones as a refreshing and guilt-free dessert option.

LOW-FAT APPLE CIDER VINEGAR CAKE

SERVES 4

INGREDIENTS

- 1½ cups all-purpose/plain flour
- 1 tsp baking soda
- ½ tsp salt
- ½ tsp ground cinnamon
- ¼ tsp ground nutmeg
- ½ cup unsweetened apple sauce
- ½ cup granulated sugar
- ¼ cup brown sugar
- 2 tbsp apple cider vinegar
- 1 tsp vanilla extract
- ½ cup low-fat milk or milk substitute

METHOD

1. Preheat the oven to 350°F (175°C). Grease and flour a baking pan.
2. In a large bowl, whisk together the flour, baking soda, salt, cinnamon, and nutmeg.
3. In a separate bowl, mix together the apple sauce, granulated sugar, brown sugar, apple cider vinegar, vanilla extract, and milk.
4. Gradually add the dry ingredients to the wet ingredients and stir until well combined.
5. Pour the batter into the prepared baking pan.
6. Bake for about 25 - 30 minutes, or until a toothpick inserted into the center comes out clean.
7. Allow the cake to cool on a rack before serving.

Healthy Snacks

APPLE CIDER VINEGAR CHOCOLATE CAKE

SERVES 4

INGREDIENTS

- 1¾ cups all-purpose/plain flour
- ¾ cup cocoa powder
- 1½ tsp baking powder
- 1½ tsp baking soda
- ½ tsp salt
- 2 large eggs
- 1 cup coconut or granulated sugar
- ½ cup vegetable oil
- 1 cup buttermilk
- ¼ cup apple cider vinegar
- 1 tsp vanilla extract
- Chocolate ganache or frosting of your choice

METHOD

1. Preheat the oven to 350°F (175°C) and grease a cake pan.
2. In a bowl, whisk together the flour, cocoa powder, baking powder, baking soda, and salt.
3. In a separate large bowl, beat the eggs and sugar until light and fluffy.
4. Add the vegetable oil, buttermilk, apple cider vinegar, and vanilla extract to the egg mixture. Mix well.
5. Gradually add the dry ingredients to the wet ingredients, mixing until just combined.
6. Pour the batter into the greased cake pan and smooth the top.
7. Bake for about 25 - 30 minutes, or until a toothpick inserted into the center comes out clean.
8. Allow the cake to cool before serving.

APPLE CRUMBLE

SERVES 4

INGREDIENTS

- 4 cups peeled and sliced apples
- 2 tbsp apple cider vinegar
- ¼ cup brown sugar
- ½ tsp ground cinnamon
- ½ cup rolled oats
- ¼ cup all-purpose/plain flour
- ¼ cup granulated sugar
- ¼ cup cold butter, diced
- Low fat or fat-free Greek yogurt for serving (optional)

METHOD

1. Preheat the oven to 375°F (190°C).
2. In a bowl, combine the sliced apples, apple cider vinegar, brown sugar, and cinnamon. Mix well to coat the apples.
3. In a separate bowl, combine the rolled oats, flour, granulated sugar, and cold butter. Mix with your fingers until crumbly.
4. Spread the apple mixture in a baking dish and sprinkle the crumble topping over it.
5. Bake for 30 - 35 minutes or until the apples are tender and the topping is golden brown.
6. Serve warm with low-fat or Greek yogurt, if desired.

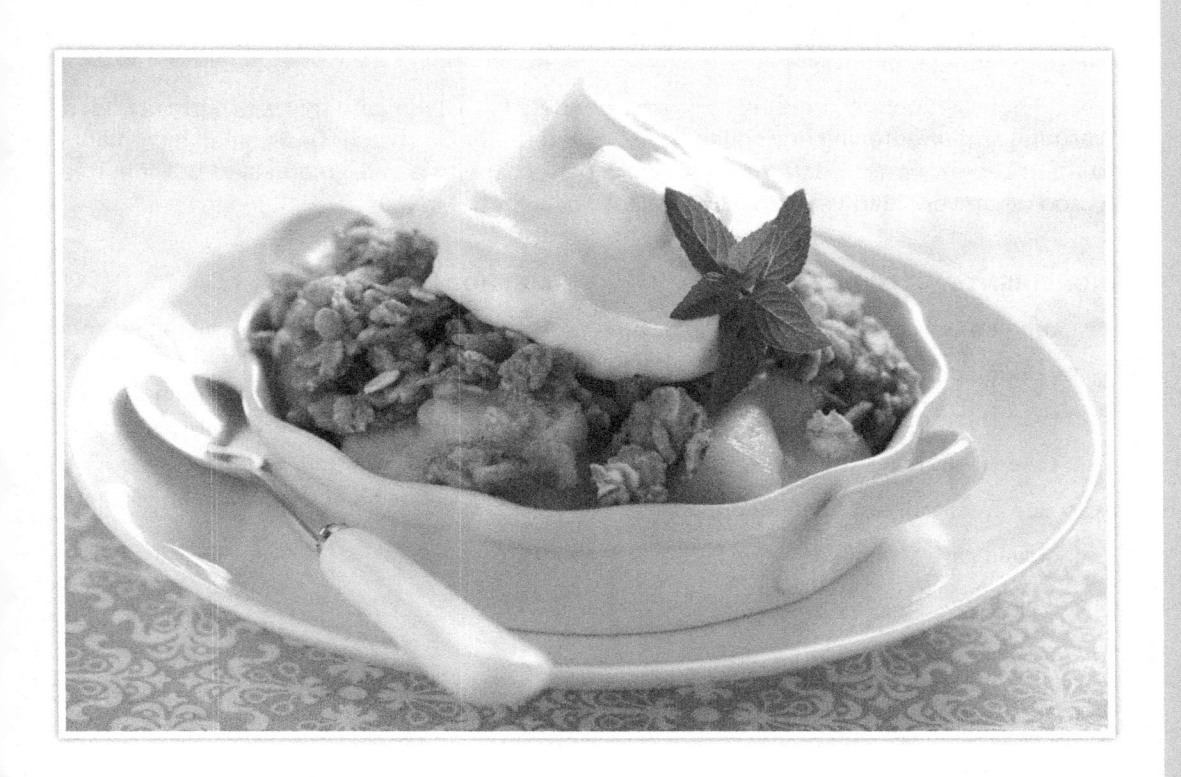

BASIC APPLE CIDER VINAIGRETTE

This vinaigrette should work with almost every salad you choose to make; simply add to your favorite salad or vegetables for a tasty, refreshing flavor that you will love.

You can alter how much garlic or honey you add to achieve the taste you want, but the following measurements will give you a balanced, even taste that is just the right combination of sweet and savory.

INGREDIENTS

- 1 cup olive oil
- ⅓ cup apple cider vinegar
- 3 tbsp honey
- 3 cloves garlic, minced
- ½ tsp black pepper
- Pinch of salt

METHOD

1. Add the vinegar to a bowl and slowly add the olive oil, whisking well as you do to emulsify the two for a smooth result.
2. Add the honey, garlic, pepper, and salt and whisk well until all the ingredients are completely blended.
3. Refrigerate for at least 30 minutes before use. A quick whisk before serving will combine all the flavors again.

HONEY MUSTARD DRESSING

A good honey-mustard dressing can work wonders for a salad and this one certainly does. Warming and sweetening any collection of mixed leaves, from your basic salad ingredients to the more exotic concoctions. This works perfectly with an all-green salad but feel free to add whatever salad vegetables you want.

INGREDIENTS

- 1 cup sunflower oil
- 1½ cups apple cider vinegar
- 3 tbsp Dijon mustard
- 2 tbsp honey
- ½ cup fresh chives, finely chopped
- 2 cloves garlic, minced
- ½ cup lemon juice
- Pinch salt

METHOD

1. In a large bowl, combine all ingredients well, reserving the olive oil.
2. Slowly whisk the olive oil into the mixture, whisking very well to ensure a smooth result.
3. Refrigerate for at least 30 minutes before serving.

ITALIAN HERB DRESSING

This works best with a big well-rounded salad so add filling vegetables such as avocado, cucumber, even chunks of boiled or steamed potatoes. Whatever you add to the salad, coat with this dressing, and enjoy!

INGREDIENTS

- 1 cup olive oil
- ¾ cup apple cider vinegar
- ½ cup fresh basil leaves, roughly chopped
- 1 tsp dried oregano
- 1 tsp garlic salt
- 1 tbsp Dijon mustard
- 4 garlic cloves, minced

METHOD

1. In a large bowl, whisk together the ingredients, reserving the oil and basil.
2. Slowly whisk the oil into the mixture, whisking well to get a smooth result as the oil and vinegar combine.
3. Stir in the chopped basil and refrigerate for at least 30 minutes before serving.

All the apple cider vinegar salad dressings above can be used over just about any salad you care to make.

Finding a salad dressing you love (especially one that incorporates healthy ingredients such as apple cider vinegar) is such a boost to your weight loss plans; it means you can incorporate new ingredients that you might not have used before. It also means that you don't get bored; you can add whatever you want and know that you will be enjoying a healthy, filling meal.

Remember that even though these dressings do contain ACV, they also include oils which can increase your daily calorie intake dramatically if not used in moderation, so don't go mad with the dressing... just enough to give a thin even coating to everything is the general rule.

If there's a lot left in the salad bowl after serving, then you've added too much!

If you want to try out some new and exciting salads that incorporate apple cider vinegar and bring a real dash of flavor to your dining table, try some of these...

RICE AND BEAN SPROUT SALAD

SERVES 3-4

INGREDIENTS

- 1 packet microwaveable wholegrain rice
- 1 tin pineapple chunks in juice, drained
- 4 scallions (green onions), finely chopped
- 50g pine nuts
- 6 radishes, finely sliced
- ½ bag of bean sprouts
- 1 tin tuna, drained (optional)

DRESSING

- 1 tbsp sunflower oil
- 1 tbsp apple cider vinegar
- Juice of 1 lime
- 1 tsp grated ginger root
- Salt and pepper to taste

METHOD

1. Cook the rice and then place in a bowl to cool.
2. Combine the pineapple chunks, scallions, pine nuts, radishes, bean sprouts and tuna if using to the cooled rice.
3. In a separate bowl add the oil, apple cider vinegar, lime juice, ginger and seasoning and mix well.
4. Add the dressing to the salad and fold in carefully using a large metal spoon.
5. Serve immediately or refrigerate until required.

TOMATO, CUCUMBER AND MINT SALAD WITH YOGURT DRESSING

SERVES 3-4

INGREDIENTS

- 6 small tomatoes, cut into chunks and cores removed
- ½ cucumber, peeled and diced
- ½ cup mint leaves
- 1 tbsp lime juice

DRESSING

- 2 tbsp low-fat yogurt
- 1 tsp grated lime rind
- 1 tbsp lime juice
- 1 tbsp apple cider vinegar
- 1 tsp grated ginger

METHOD

1. Place tomatoes, cucumber, and mint in a serving bowl.
2. Drizzle over with some of the lime juice and put into the fridge whilst preparing the dressing.
3. To make the dressing place the yogurt, lime juice, apple cider vinegar, lime rind and grated ginger into a bowl and mix well.
4. The dressing can be either drizzled over the salad or served separately.

CRAB AND PAPAYA SALAD

SERVES 2

INGREDIENTS

- 1 dressed crab or 1 tin of crab in brine, drained
- 1 large papaya, diced
- 80g packet of herb salad or mixed salad leaves
- Freshly ground black pepper

DRESSING

- 1 tbsp olive oil
- 4 tsp lime juice
- 1½ tsp freshly grated ginger
- 1 tsp light soy sauce
- 1 tbsp apple cider vinegar
- 4 scallions finely chopped

METHOD

1. Firstly make the dressing by combining all the ingredients together and mix thoroughly.
2. Just before serving gently combine the crab and papaya into the dressing and season with black pepper.
3. Arrange the salad leaves on a plate and top with the crab mixture.

WARM LENTIL SALAD WITH PARMA HAM, CHICKEN AND ROCKET

SERVES 4

INGREDIENTS

- 1 red onion, halved and very finely sliced
- Handful flat leaf parsley, roughly chopped
- 4 ripe tomatoes, roughly chopped
- 2 tsp small capers, drained
- 250g pouch ready cooked puy lentils
- 8 slices Parma ham
- 2 cooked chicken breasts, skin removed, torn into pieces
- 100g wild rocket

DRESSING

- 1 tbsp apple cider vinegar
- 1 tbsp olive oil
- Salt and pepper

METHOD

1. Put the onion in a bowl, drizzle over the vinegar, then season with salt and pepper. Set aside for 10 minutes or so until the onion has softened slightly.
2. Meanwhile, in another large bowl mix the parsley with the tomatoes and capers.
3. When ready to serve, tip the lentils into a sieve and rinse with boiling water from the kettle, drain.
4. Toss the onions and their juices into the lentils, add the olive oil, and carefully mix everything together.
5. Spoon onto a large serving platter and top with the chicken, ham, and rocket.

BEAN, POTATO AND TUNA SALAD

SERVES 4

INGREDIENTS

- 300g new potatoes, cut into chunks
- 175g green beans, trimmed and halved
- 175g tinned butter beans
- 1 can tuna in water, drained well
- Good handful rocket or watercress leaves

DRESSING

- 2 tsp harissa paste
- 1 tbsp apple cider vinegar
- 1 tbsp olive oil
- Salt and pepper

METHOD

1. Put the potatoes in a pan of boiling water and cook for 6 – 8 minutes until almost tender.
2. Add both types of beans and cook for a further 5 mins until everything is cooked.
3. Meanwhile, make the dressing. Whisk together the harissa and vinegar in a small bowl with a little seasoning.
4. Whisk in the oil until the dressing is thickened.
5. Drain potatoes well and toss with half the dressing, then leave to cool.
6. Flake the tuna, then fold into the potatoes along with the beans. Add the remaining dressing then gently toss.
7. Divide into four bowls and serve each portion with a handful of rocket or watercress.

MINT SAUCE

MULTIPLE SERVINGS

INGREDIENTS

- Bunch of fresh mint, removed from stalks and finely chopped
- 5 tbsp boiling water
- 3 tbsp apple cider vinegar
- 2 tbsp malt vinegar
- 1 tbsp fruit sugar/stevia or coconut sugar
- Pinch of salt

METHOD

1. Wash and finely chop the fresh mint, then add to a small bowl.
2. Next add the apple cider vinegar, malt vinegar, boiling water, sugar, and a pinch of salt.
3. Mix together well and add to your favorite meals.

Here are some common dishes and foods that mint sauce can be used with:

Lamb: Mint sauce is often served as a condiment with roasted or grilled lamb dishes. The cool, refreshing flavor of mint complements the rich taste of lamb.

Roast vegetables: Mint sauce can be drizzled over roasted vegetables, such as roasted potatoes or carrots, to add a fresh and tangy flavor.

Salads: Mint sauce can be used as a dressing or a flavoring component in various salads, particularly those that include fruits, such as watermelon or citrus salads.

Samosas and other Indian snacks: In Indian cuisine, mint sauce, often referred to as mint chutney, is a popular accompaniment to snacks like samosas, pakoras, or kebabs. It adds a refreshing contrast to the savory and spicy flavors of these dishes.

Middle Eastern dishes: Mint sauce is commonly used in Middle Eastern cuisine. It can be served with dishes like falafel, grilled meats, tabbouleh salad, or as a dipping sauce for flatbreads.

Roast meats: In addition to lamb, mint sauce can also be served with other roasted meats, such as roast beef or roast chicken, as a complementary sauce or condiment.

APPLE CIDER VINEGAR DRINKS

Apple Cider Vinegar and Water

This is the simplest and most common way to consume ACV. Mix one to two tablespoons of ACV with a glass of water (8-16 ounces). You can adjust the ratio to suit your taste preferences. Some people also add a squeeze of lemon juice or a teaspoon of honey to enhance the flavor.

ACV Detox Drink

This drink combines ACV with other ingredients known for their potential health benefits. One common recipe includes mixing two tablespoons of ACV, two tablespoons of lemon juice, one teaspoon of honey, a pinch of cayenne pepper, and a cup of water. This drink is often consumed in the morning on an empty stomach.

ACV and Green Tea

Brew a cup of green or herbal tea and let it cool slightly. Mix in one to two tablespoons of ACV and optionally add a squeeze of lemon or a teaspoon of honey for added flavor. Be sure to choose herbal tea that does not contain any added sweeteners or calories.

ACV and Fruit Infused Water

Create a refreshing and flavored ACV drink by infusing water with fruits and herbs. Slice fruits like oranges, strawberries, or apples, and add them to a pitcher of water along with a few tablespoons of ACV. Allow the mixture to infuse in the refrigerator for a few hours before consuming.

ACV Smoothie

Incorporate ACV into your favorite smoothie recipe. Blend together fruits, leafy greens, a liquid of your choice (such as almond milk or coconut water) and add a tablespoon of ACV for an extra nutritional boost.

ACV Shot

If you prefer a quick and concentrated method for taking your ACV each day, you can take a straight shot of ACV. Measure out one to two tablespoons of ACV and consume it in one go. Follow this immediately with a glass of water or rinse your mouth out well afterwards to protect your tooth enamel.

NOTE

Remember to start with smaller amounts of ACV and gradually increase the quantity to allow your body to adjust. It's important to listen to your body and discontinue its use if you experience any adverse reactions. Consulting with a healthcare professional can also provide personalized advice based on your specific health needs.

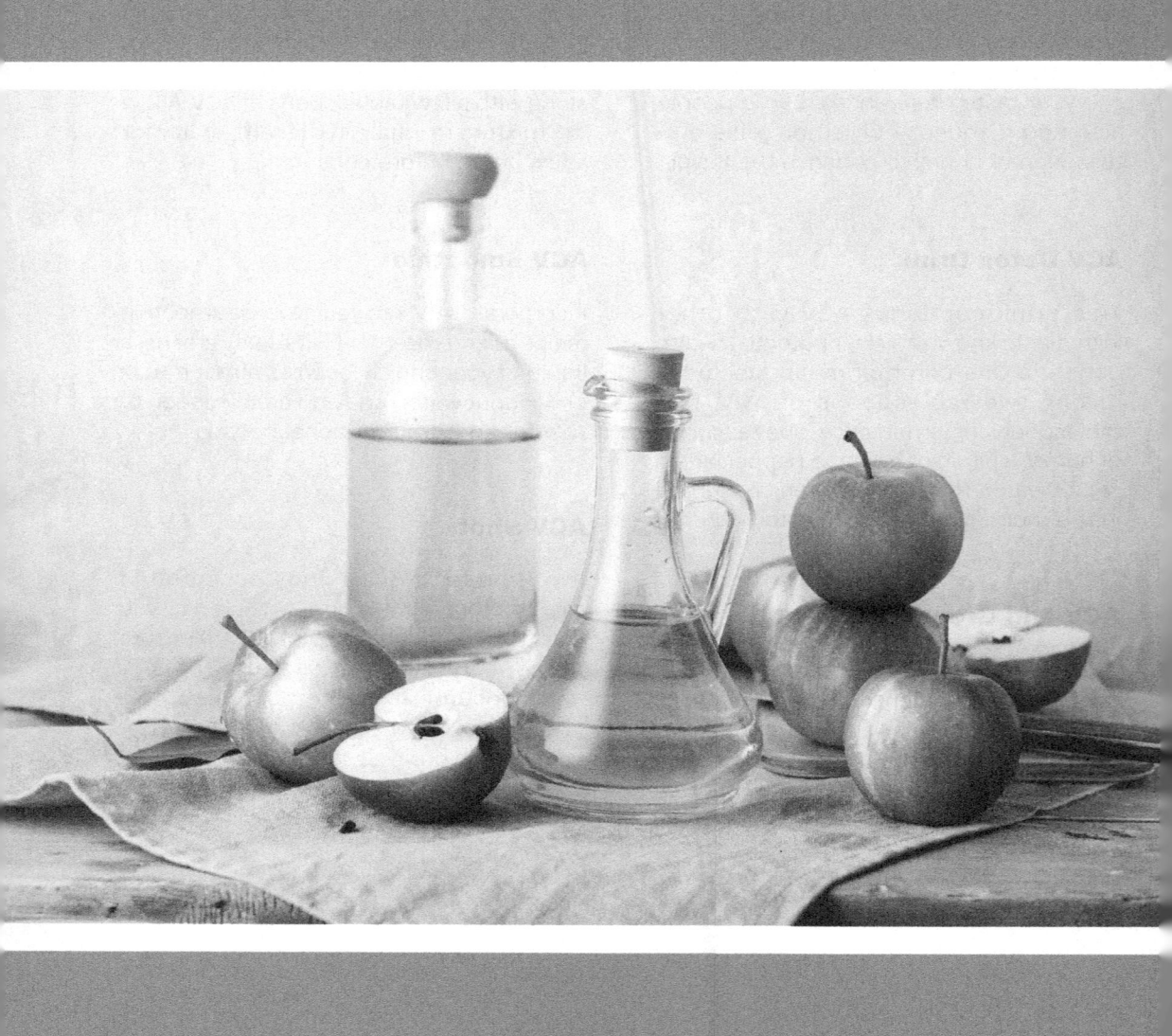

APPLE CIDER VINEGAR FREQUENTLY ASKED QUESTIONS

> "The best way to lose weight and make a lasting change to your life is to make small, consistent changes to the things you eat and drink. Don't try and go all in. If you deny yourself everything you love, your mind will rebel and you'll be fighting against it every minute of every day"

Q. How much apple cider vinegar should I use?

A. The appropriate amount of apple cider vinegar (ACV) to use can vary depending on factors such as your health goals, tolerance, and the specific purpose for which you are using it. Here are some general recommendations:

1. Diluted ACV for general health and well-being: Start by mixing 1-2 tablespoons of ACV with a glass of water (8-16 ounces). You can adjust the amount of ACV to suit your taste preferences and tolerance. It's generally advisable to start with a smaller amount and gradually increase it if desired.

2. ACV for weight management: Some studies have suggested that consuming 1-2 tablespoons of ACV before meals may help with appetite control and weight management. However, it's important to note that the evidence is limited, and individual responses can vary. If using ACV for weight management, you can try taking a tablespoon or two before meals, diluted with water.

3. ACV for specific health conditions or concerns: If you are using ACV for a specific health condition, it's best to consult with a healthcare professional for personalized advice. They can guide you on the appropriate dosage based on your specific needs and any underlying health conditions you may have.

It's worth noting that while ACV is generally considered safe for most people, consuming excessive amounts, or using it improperly can have negative effects. It's important to listen to your body and adjust the amount of ACV according to your tolerance and any potential side effects you may experience. If you have any concerns or questions, it's always a good idea to consult with a healthcare professional for guidance.

Q. Why do you need to dilute apple cider vinegar?

A. Diluting apple cider vinegar (ACV) with water is typically recommended for a few reasons:

1. Reducing acidity: ACV is highly acidic, and undiluted vinegar can be harsh on tooth enamel, your throat, and the delicate tissues of the digestive system. Diluting ACV with water helps lower the acidity and minimize the potential for irritation or damage.

2. Protecting tooth enamel: The acidity of undiluted ACV can erode tooth enamel over time, leading to dental problems such as tooth sensitivity and increased vulnerability to cavities. By diluting ACV, you can reduce its direct contact with teeth and minimize the risk of damage to tooth enamel. It's also advised to rinse your mouth with water or brush your teeth after consuming ACV to further protect tooth enamel.

3. Reducing digestive discomfort: Consuming undiluted ACV may cause discomfort in the digestive system, such as burning sensations or upset stomach, due to its high acidity. Diluting ACV with water can help make it more tolerable and gentler on the digestive tract.

4. Easier consumption: ACV has a strong and tangy taste, which some people find unpleasant when consumed on its own. Diluting it with water can make it more palatable and easier to consume.

The recommended ratio for diluting ACV can vary, but a common guideline is to mix one to two tablespoons of ACV with a glass of water (8-16 ounces). However, personal preferences and tolerances may vary, so you can adjust the ratio to suit your taste.

It's important to note that even when diluted, ACV may still cause discomfort or adverse effects in some individuals. If you experience any negative reactions or have concerns, it's advisable to consult with a healthcare professional.

Q. What are the main problems with taking apple cider vinegar?

A. While apple cider vinegar (ACV) is generally considered safe for consumption, there are a few potential problems or considerations to be aware of:

1. Tooth enamel erosion: ACV is highly acidic, and consuming undiluted ACV or using it frequently without proper dilution can erode tooth enamel over time. To minimize this risk, it's recommended to dilute ACV with water and rinse your mouth with water or brush your teeth afterwards.

2. Digestive issues: Some individuals may experience digestive discomfort, such as heartburn, stomach upset, or nausea, when consuming ACV - especially if it's consumed in large amounts or on an empty stomach. If you have a history of gastrointestinal issues, it's advisable to exercise caution and start with small amounts of ACV to assess your tolerance.

3. Interaction with medications: ACV may interact with certain medications, including diuretics, insulin, and potassium-lowering medications. It's important to consult with a healthcare professional if you are taking medications to ensure that ACV will not interfere with their effectiveness or cause any adverse effects.

4. Delayed stomach emptying: ACV has been found to slow down stomach

emptying, which can affect individuals with gastroparesis or delayed gastric emptying. If you have this condition or any other gastrointestinal disorders, it's recommended to seek medical advice before starting to consume ACV.

5. Allergic reactions: Some individuals may be allergic to apples or develop allergic reactions to ACV. If you have known apple allergies or experience any allergic symptoms like hives, itching, or swelling, discontinue the use of ACV and seek medical attention.

It's important to note that the scientific evidence supporting the benefits and risks of ACV is limited, and individual experiences may vary. It's always a good idea to consult with a healthcare professional before incorporating ACV into your daily routine, especially if you have underlying health conditions or concerns. They can provide personalized guidance based on your specific needs and help you make informed decisions about its use.

Q. How long does apple cider vinegar last once opened?

A. The shelf life of apple cider vinegar (ACV) can vary depending on factors such as storage conditions and the presence of additives or preservatives. Generally, if stored properly, ACV can maintain its quality for an extended period of time. Here are some guidelines:

Unopened ACV: Unopened bottles of ACV can typically last for an indefinite period when stored in a cool, dark place such as a pantry. It is best to refer to the expiration date on the bottle for guidance.

Opened ACV: Once the bottle is opened, ACV can remain usable for a long time, but its quality may gradually decline over time. To maximize its shelf life, it's important to store it properly. Keep the ACV tightly sealed in its original bottle and store it in a cool, dark place away from direct sunlight and heat. Exposure to air, light, and heat can accelerate the deterioration of ACV. If stored properly, opened ACV can maintain its quality for several months to a year or even longer.

Signs of spoilage: Over time, ACV may undergo some changes such as sedimentation or discoloration. These changes are usually harmless and can be remedied by shaking the bottle before use. However, if you notice significant changes in color, texture, or smell, or if mould or signs of fermentation develop, it is best to discard the ACV as it may have spoiled.

Q. What can I do If I don't like the taste of apple cider vinegar?

A. If you don't enjoy the taste of apple cider vinegar (ACV), there are a few strategies you can try to incorporate it into your routine:

1. Dilute it: Mix a tablespoon or two of ACV with a larger amount of water. Start with a higher water-to-ACV ratio and gradually decrease the dilution as you become accustomed to the taste. You can also add a splash of honey or a squeeze of lemon to enhance the flavor.

2. Use it in recipes: Incorporate ACV into your meals by using it as an ingredient in salad dressings, marinades, or sauces. Combined with other flavors, the taste of ACV may become less noticeable.

3. Take it as a shot: If diluting ACV doesn't work for you, you can try taking a quick shot of undiluted ACV followed by a glass of water or a flavored beverage

to help mask the taste. Be sure to rinse your mouth afterwards to protect your tooth enamel due to the high acidity of ACV.

4. Consider ACV capsules or pills: ACV is also available in capsule or pill form, which eliminates the taste entirely. These supplements allow you to reap the potential benefits of ACV without having to consume the liquid.

5. Experiment with flavored options: Some brands offer flavored ACV varieties, such as honey-infused or fruit-flavored options. These can provide a more palatable taste while still providing the benefits of ACV.

6. Mask it with a sweeter taste: If you find that ACV doesn't suit your taste preferences at all, you can try taking it in fruit juice. For example, pure apple, pineapple, or orange juice may mask the taste enough for you to be able to drink it comfortably.

BOOK SUMMARY

Well, that's it, thanks for reading, I hope you've gained something from my experience and knowledge.

I just want to quickly recap what you should have learnt from this book.

In section 1, I discuss all about apple cider vinegar and give you a compelling argument for giving it a go. We discuss its uses for general health as well as for weight loss. I give you a recipe so you can actually make your own ACV and we look at the most recent research into the benefits of ACV has on weight loss.

In section 2, I give you three methods for using ACV as a tool for losing weight…

First, we look at simply adding it to your diet, by drinking an ACV mixture before each meal.

Secondly, we consider its use as part of a 7-day detox.

Thirdly, I show you how you can include ACV into a healthy weight loss diet which you can use over the long term.

In the last section, we look at how you can add walking into your day to get even more from your weight loss efforts, and I give you over 40 different meal and snack ideas which all include apple cider vinegar.

Finally, we look at how you can use ACV in the home or as part of a beauty routine and I give you some charts and logs, so you can both plan and monitor your progress as you go along.

ABOUT THE AUTHOR

Please allow me to introduce myself. My name is Jago Holmes, and I am the author and creator of "*The Apple Cider Vinegar Weight Loss Revolution*," a book all about the many ways to use one of the oldest and most well-known dietary supplements in the world to help you lose weight. I am also the owner and principal trainer here at New Image Personal Training in Halifax, UK. We regularly work with over 100 clients every week in our exclusive 1:1 studio.

I am a fully qualified and experienced fitness trainer and weight loss expert. My personal training company has been in operation for more than 20 years now and we consistently get great results with our clients, and so I'd like to share my knowledge and success with you now.

I've written hundreds of magazine articles as well as countless blogs and numerous website posts and created a range of digital e-books and weight loss packages. I regularly presented fat loss seminars as well as running my acclaimed *8 Week Weight Loss Challenge*.

I studied at the University of Leeds, completing my training with the YMCA in 2000. After three years, I attained the YMCA Personal Trainer Award - one of the highest and most respected qualifications available in the UK for Personal Trainers.

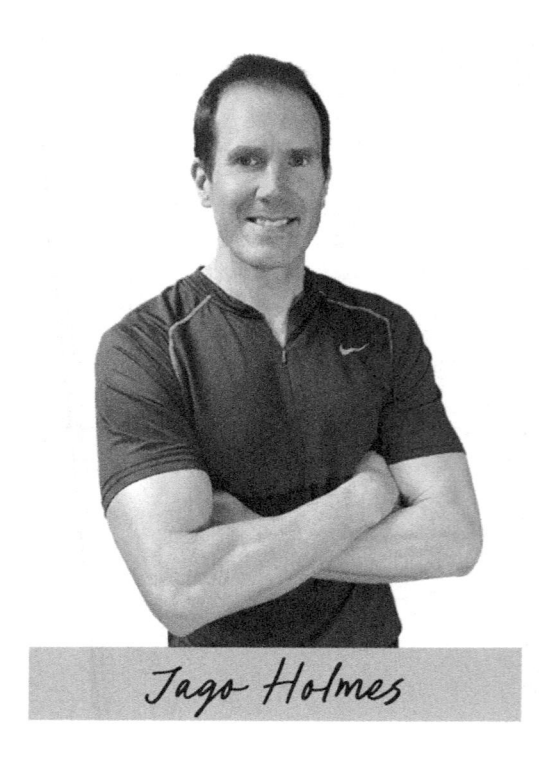

Jago Holmes

I have a lifetime love and passion for all things related to health and fitness and this helps me to think 'outside the box' in search of solutions to many of my client's most challenging situations.

Lack of time, medical conditions, food intolerances, lack of motivation, unusual working patterns, limited budgets... you name it, and the chances are I have worked with a client who had that same problem.

As a result of this, I have created a range of books that address many of these needs and more.

It's amazing how one piece of knowledge, clever tip or trick can literally change someone's life around - instantly transforming the way they think about their own circumstances. I like to look for answers from outside of the usual places that most people search.

What I've tried to do with my books is write in an easy-to-understand way that answers the questions that people need without being blinded by science.

My books are not meant for academics or boffins, they're meant to be read and understood by everyday people. I try to add unusual or little-known techniques into what I write that people can use because they have been proven to be effective in all manner of ways.

Often, we look to the most obvious answers to losing weight... eating less and exercising more, and, whilst this is certainly the answer in many cases, sometimes there are other issues present and things that can be done differently.

In my writing, this is what I'm looking for - ways of doing things differently and more effectively that can make a real difference to people's lives.

I hope you enjoy reading my work and put into action the steps, techniques, tips, and advice that you learn. If you like what you've read and think others would also benefit, then please

leave your positive comments for others to read about your experience, as it makes the Amazon marketplace a much more honest and enjoyable place for people to shop and buy books.

If you can think of any ways you feel this book could be improved, please send an email to me – *jago@jagoholmes.com* and I'll try to add your suggestions.

To your health and fitness

Jago Holmes CPT

Personal Trainer and Weight Loss Expert

OTHER BOOKS THAT MIGHT BE OF INTEREST TO YOU

Walking For Weight Loss

A fantastic weight loss walking program with four unique and HIGHLY effective walking techniques is the easiest and most effective way to blast through stubborn fat stores at the fastest rate possible. With a range of five different plans to follow, you're sure to find the perfect solution for you.

This book is designed to help anyone lose weight. *It's an effective alternative for those who don't want to use a gym/fitness class or hate the idea of going running etc.*

Go here to find out more about a unique fat burning system you can start today –
https://www.amazon.com/dp/B0C53WR3G4

5K Training for Beginners

If you've ever fancied running a 5k or just getting fit enough to run 5 kilometers in one go (that's a little over 3 miles to you and me!) and you want to do it in the shortest amount of time, without risking injury, boredom or losing interest, then this book is for you.

5k Training for Beginners - From Couch to 5k Runner In 8 Weeks or Less, contains **everything you need to know about running a 5k** in the fastest, most efficient, and fun way.

Go here to order your copy today –
https://www.amazon.com/dp/B0085VG4IO

USEFUL FORMS, PLANNERS AND LOGS

Aims and Objectives

Four Week / Short Term Aims

AIM #1
AIM #2
AIM #3
AIM #4
To Achieve This, I Will:

Twelve Week / Mid Term Aims

AIM #1
AIM #2
AIM #3
AIM #4
To Achieve This, I Will:

Long Term Aims

AIM #1
AIM #2
AIM #3
AIM #4
To Achieve This, I Will:

NOTES

WEEKLY MEASUREMENTS

How to Use This Form

Whenever you set out on a journey it is important that you chart your progress regularly. Jumping on the scales every day certainly isn't productive, but I would recommend that you do this once a week and take your measurements at the same time.

You should use your hips and waist measurements and not your weight to assess whether progress is being made. By taking measurements at regular intervals, you are doing two things. Firstly, you can see whether your current efforts are having effect, if they are, then keep doing what you are doing- if not make some changes. For example, you might be able to increase the amount of activity you are doing.

Secondly it maintains your awareness and helps to keep you focused on your goals and objectives.

DATE	WEIGHT	WAIST	HIPS

Start your measurements on week 1. Take them at the same time and on the same day each week. Measure around the narrowest part of your waist and the widest part of your hips.

Your Workout Log

DATE:	TRAINING TIME:	DAY:

Vital Statistics	
Resting Heart Rate Before:	
Weight:	
Sleep in Hours the Night Before:	
Eaten Well Through the Day:	
Workout Type:	**Overall Difficulty Level (1-10):**
Distance:	
Course:	
Duration:	
Average Heart Rate:	**End Heart Rate:**
Weather:	**Temperature:**
Mood and Enjoyment	
Hated it:	
Felt Great:	
Really Enjoyed it:	
Was OK:	

NOTES

You can use this form to monitor your workouts and chart your progress. You may want to use all the sections on the form or just a few. Whatever you do decide, just make sure that you keep a record of your sessions. This will help motivate you to do more in the future and perhaps more importantly, reinforce the fact that what you've done in the past is helping you to get fitter.

I suggest that you copy this page and print one out for each session you do.

Activity Planner

Plan your activities in advance, choose things you enjoy. Aim to do some form of activity at least 5 times a week.

WEEKS	MONDAY	TUESDAY	WEDNESDAY	THURSDAY	FRIDAY	SATURDAY	SUNDAY
4							
3							
2							
1							

Made in the USA
Las Vegas, NV
18 September 2023